PEDIATRICS

MEDICAL EXAMINATION REVIEW

PEDIATRICS

Seventh Edition, Volume 11

650 Multiple-Choice Questions
with Referenced, Explanatory Answers

Victor A. LaCerva, M.D., F.A.A.P.

Clinical Assistant Professor
Department of Pediatrics
University of New Mexico Medical Center
District Health Officer, District II
New Mexico

MEDICAL EXAMINATION PUBLISHING COMPANY

Medical Examination Publishing Company
A Division of
Elsevier Science Publishing Co., Inc.
52 Vanderbilt Avenue, New York, New York 10017

Library of Congress Cataloging in Publication Data

Main entry under title:

Medical examination review.
    Includes various editions of some volumes.
    Includes bibliographical references.
    1. Medicine – Examinations, questions, etc.
RC5.M4   610'.76   61-66847
ISBN 0-444-01036-X

Current printing (last digit)
10 9 8 7 6 5 4

Manufactured in the United States of America

*This book acknowledges teachers everywhere,
for their wisdom, vision, and patience.*

*It is dedicated to my father and grandfather,
who have been my teachers
in more ways than they realize.*

Contents

Preface

The seventh edition of *Medical Examination Review, Volume 11, Pediatrics*, has been substantially revised and updated to keep in step with current trends in medical education and the continuing expansion of scientific knowledge. It is designed to help you prepare for course examinations, National Boards Part II, the Federation Licensing Examination (FLEX), and examinations for foreign medical graduates.

The range of subjects included in this volume is based on the content outline of the National Board of Medical Examiners, which develops the question pool for the tests mentioned above, and reflects the scope and depth of what is taught in medical schools today. The questions themselves are organized in broad categories to give you a representative sampling of the material covered in course work, while helping you define those general areas to which you need to devote attention. For your convenience in selective study, the answers (with commentary and references) follow each section of questions.

Each question has been scrutinized by specialists to verify that it is relevant and current. The author's care in item construction gives you questions that will provide good practice in familiarizing yourself with the format of objective-type tests. Questions of each type—one best response, matching, multiple, true-false, and so on—are grouped together. They are modeled as closely as possible after those used by the Board.

Using this book, you may identify areas of strength and weakness in your own command of the subject. Specific references to widely used textbooks allow you to return to the authoritative source for further study. This volume supplements the lettered answers with brief explanations intended to prompt you to think about the choices (correct and incorrect), to put the answers in broadened perspective, and to add to your fund of knowledge. The questions and answers, taken together, emphasize problem solving and application of underlying principles as well as retention of factual knowledge.

1 Perinatology

DIRECTIONS: Each of the questions or incomplete statements below is followed by five suggested answers or completions. Select the **one** that is best in each case.

1. At birth the blood volume is approximately
   A. 65 ml/kg body weight
   B. 85 ml/kg body weight
   C. 110 ml/kg body weight
   D. 125 ml/kg body weight
   E. 150 ml/kg body weight

2. All of the following may be sources of blood in the vomitus of a two-day-old newborn EXCEPT
   A. placental blood swallowed at delivery
   B. suctioning
   C. breastfeeding
   D. irritation caused by silver nitrate
   E. gastrointestinal hemorrhage

3. The APT test is used for what purpose?
   A. Crude test for carbon monoxide poisoning
   B. Semiquantitative test for lead poisoning
   C. Qualitative test for fetal hemoglobin
   D. Screening test for S hemoglobin
   E. Test for blood viscosity

1

4. Therapy for neonatal necrotizing enterocolitis may include all of the following EXCEPT
   A. systemic antibiotics
   B. surgical resection
   C. discontinuance of oral feeding
   D. correction of low blood volume
   E. use of elemental enteral feedings

5. Meconium ileus in the newborn is best treated by
   A. enzyme replacement
   B. barium enema
   C. surgery
   D. irrigation of the gut with N-acetylcysteine
   E. phosphate enema

6. All of the following statements are true concerning serum transport of bilirubin EXCEPT
   A. it is transported primarily bound to albumin
   B. sulfonamides compete for binding sites
   C. one mole of albumin can bind approximately one mole of bilirubin in vivo
   D. multiple binding sites exist
   E. the first binding site has greatest affinity

7. Craniotabes may be present in all of the following EXCEPT
   A. premature infants
   B. rickets
   C. hydrocephalus
   D. normal infants
   E. the neonate showing signs of syphilis

8. Polyhydramnios is frequently associated with fetal malformations, including
   A. renal agenesis
   B. anencephaly
   C. pulmonary hypoplasia
   D. urethral atresia
   E. amnion nodosum

9. Mongolian spots are characterized by all of the following EXCEPT
   A. they are permanent
   B. they are usually of a slate blue pigmentation
   C. they are generally observed over the buttocks
   D. the area of pigmentation is well demarcated
   E. they are not associated with trisomy syndromes

10. All of the following physical signs may be useful in estimating gestational age at birth EXCEPT
    A. there are only one or two transverse skin creases on the sole of the foot until 36 weeks of gestation
    B. the breast nodule is usually not palpable at 33 or 34 weeks
    C. the breast nodule is usually 4 to 10 mm in term infants
    D. the testes are descending and rugae cover the entire scrotal surface by 34 weeks
    E. the texture of scalp hair

11. Caput succedaneum is characterized by all of the following EXCEPT
    A. a diffuse, edematous swelling of the soft tissues of the scalp, involving the portion presenting during vertex delivery
    B. it may extend across the midline
    C. it may extend across suture lines
    D. edema usually disappears within two to three months
    E. the scalp overlying the area may show mild bruising

12. A newborn exhibits respiratory distress, distension of neck veins, low blood pressure, hyperresonance, diminished breath sounds over one side of the chest, and subcutaneous emphysema. The most likely diagnosis is
    A. hyaline membrane disease
    B. staphylococcal pneumonia
    C. pneumothorax and pneumomediastinum
    D. primary atelectasis
    E. diaphragmatic hernia

13. In a newborn with oral moniliasis, the most common primary source of infection is
    A. maternal source (vaginal)
    B. contaminated fomites
    C. following use of AgNO₃
    D. contact by hospital carriers
    E. systemic antibiotic therapy

14. Meconium impaction is associated with
    A. cretinism
    B. cystic fibrosis
    C. thrush
    D. hyaline membrane disease
    E. trisomy 21 syndrome

15. Persistent jaundice during the first month of life may be associated with all of the following EXCEPT
    A. cytomegalic inclusion disease
    B. congenital atresia of the bile ducts
    C. galactosemia
    D. Rh incompatibility
    E. penicillin treatment

Figure 1 Bilirubin levels in breastfeeding jaundice. Jaundice associated with breastfeeding is a fairly common occurrence. This illustration shows the normal course of "untreated" breast milk jaundice.

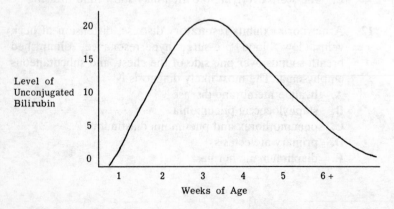

Level of Unconjugated Bilirubin

Weeks of Age

16. All of the following are characteristic of jaundice associated with breastfeeding EXCEPT (Fig. 1)
    A. significant elevations of unconjugated bilirubin
    B. a rapid fall in serum bilirubin after discontinuation of nursing
    C. nursing can be resumed after several days without return of hyperbilirubinemia
    D. significant elevations of conjugated bilirubin
    E. kernicterus has never been reported to occur as a result of breast milk jaundice alone

17. All of the following are characteristic of single umbilical artery EXCEPT
    A. presence in about five of 1000 births
    B. about one-third of such infants have congenital abnormalities
    C. trisomy 21 is frequently found
    D. among twins the rate of occurrence is 35 per 1000
    E. the associated congenital abnormalities may involve the genitourinary tract

18. All of the following are usually associated with cretinism EXCEPT
    A. constipation
    B. prolonged jaundice
    C. lethargy
    D. tetany
    E. hypotonia

19. Hypoglycemia has been observed in newborns
    A. with low birthweights and respiratory distress syndrome
    B. with anoxic injury
    C. with hypothermia
    D. who are small for gestational age
    E. with high PaO_2

DIRECTIONS: For each of the following questions or incomplete statements below, **one or more** of the answers or completions given is correct. Select

A   if only **1, 2,** and **3** are correct,
B   if only **1** and **3** are correct,
C   if only **2** and **4** are correct,
D   if only **4** is correct,
E   if all are correct.

20. Amniocentesis is useful in establishing the prenatal diagnosis of
    1.   Down syndrome
    2.   meningomyelocele
    3.   erythroblastosis fetalis
    4.   achondroplasia

21. Fetal malformations that are frequently associated with poly-hydramnios include
    1.   duodenal atresia
    2.   renal atresia
    3.   esophageal atresia
    4.   pulmonary hypoplasia

22. Maternal urine estriol determinations can be used to
    1.   ascertain gestational age of the fetus
    2.   indicate fetal growth retardation
    3.   diagnose preeclampsia
    4.   serve as an index of placental function

23. Ultrasound can be used during pregnancy to
    1.   determine crown rump length
    2.   determine fetal sex
    3.   determine the biparietal diameter
    4.   accurately determine fetal weight

24. Intrauterine fetal growth retardation may be associated with
    1. maternal drug addiction
    2. maternal smoking
    3. fetal viral infection
    4. maternal aspirin abuse

25. Gestations that produce multiple births
    1. are classified as high risk
    2. are always delivered by cesarean section
    3. can produce infants with discordance in body size at birth
    4. are not associated with the premature onset of labor

DIRECTIONS: Each group of questions below consists of five lettered headings, followed by a list of numbered words, phrases or statements. For each numbered word, phrase or statement, select the **one** lettered heading that is most closely associated with it. Each lettered heading may be selected once, more than once, or not at all.

    A. Localized edema
    B. Rectal bleeding
    C. Epstein pearls
    D. Horseshoe kidney
    E. Generalized edema

    26. Normal newborn
    27. Trisomy 18
    28. Congenital nephrosis
    29. Turner syndrome
    30. Hydrops fetalis

DIRECTIONS: This section consists of situations, each followed by a series of questions. Study each situation, and select the **one** best answer to each question following it.

CASE 1 (Questions 31–33): You are called to the nursery to examine a full-term five-pound male infant born to a G2 P1001 O positive mother. The infant has been irritable since birth earlier in the day, with poor feeding and some loose stools.

31. Differential diagnosis at this point may include each of the following EXCEPT
    A. hypoglycemia
    B. hypocalcemia
    C. neonatal narcotic withdrawal
    D. respiratory distress syndrome
    E. sepsis

32. Review of the chart indicates that the mother has a history of drug addiction, and has received little prenatal care. Signs and symptoms in the infant compatible with withdrawal syndrome include all of the following EXCEPT
    A. jitteriness
    B. diarrhea
    C. shrill cry
    D. yawning
    E. low birth weight

33. Appropriate actions in caring for this infant may include each of the following EXCEPT
    A. social service consultation
    B. close follow-up because of the possible recurrence of withdrawal symptoms
    C. intravenous therapy if needed to avoid dehydration
    D. use of phenobarb, chlorpromazine, or paregoric to control symptoms
    E. duration of therapy usually four to six weeks

CASE 2 (Questions 34–35):   You are called to the delivery room to assist at the birth of an infant suspected of being postdates. There is evidence of fetal distress with passage of meconium.

34. True statements about postmaturity include each of the following EXCEPT
    A. the infants are usually 42 to 44 weeks
    B. the fingernails and umbilical cord may be yellow stained
    C. birth weight is usually greater than the 50th percentile
    D. the placenta is of normal size
    E. there is an increased incidence of fetal distress, often with meconium aspiration

35. The infant is born without distress or evidence of meconium aspiration. He is taken to the nursery. This infant is at increased risk for all of the following EXCEPT
    A. hypoglycemia
    B. hypocalcemia
    C. birth injury
    D. polycythemia
    E. anemia

Perinatology
Answers and Comments

1. B. At birth, the blood volume is about 85 ml/kg body weight, falling to about 75 ml/kg after the first month. (Ref. 1, p. 162)

2. D. Sources other than the infant's gastrointestinal tract must be sought in the differential diagnosis of vomited blood in the neonate. Silver nitrate used as GC prophylaxis is applied directly to the conjunctivae and is not a source of blood in the vomitus. (Ref. 1, p. 922)

3. C. The APT test is useful in distinguishing maternal blood from newborn blood. (Ref. 1, p. 922)

4. E. Because of the high mortality associated with necrotizing enterocolitis, aggressive treatment should be initiated. If accompanied by shock, immediate correction is critical to survival. Elemental enteral feeding is contraindicated because of the high osmotic load it imposes on the gut. (Ref. 1, p. 959)

5. C. In older children, acetylcysteine irrigation may relieve acute obstructions. Recurrences may be prevented by increasing the dose of pancreatic enzyme supplementation. Neonates tolerate nonsurgical treatments poorly. (Ref. 1, p. 958)

6. C. The molar ratio in vivo is 1:2; 1 g of albumin can bind approximately 16 mg of bilirubin. (Ref. 1, p. 999)

7. D. It is also seen in osteogenesis imperfecta, and craniotabes present near suture lines may be normal (Ref. 2, p. 333)

8. B. The polyhydramnios associated with anencephaly may be caused by the faulty formation or excretion of antidiuretic hormone. The other conditions cited are associated with oligohydramnios. (Ref. 2, p. 330)

9. A. Mongolian spots usually disappear within the first year of life. There is no increased incidence of these lesions with the various trisomy syndromes. (Ref. 2, p. 332)

10. D. The testes are usually not completely descended until after 36 weeks and the scrotal rugae are few and limited to the anterior and inferior aspects of a relatively small scrotum. (Ref. 2, p. 343)

11. D. The edema of caput succedaneum usually disappears within the first few days of life and requires no specific therapy. (Ref. 2, p. 356)

12. C. The chest findings suggest a pneumothorax, and subcutaneous emphysema in a newborn strongly suggests pneumomediastinum. (Ref. 2, p. 438)

13. A. There is a positive correlation between maternal vaginal and infantile oral moniliasis. This is the primary means of infection in a newborn. (Ref. 2, p. 376)

14. B. Meconium ileus is associated with cystic fibrosis. Deficiency of pancreatic enzyme limits normal digestive activities in the intestine. As a result, meconium is left in a viscid mucilaginous state, and it clings to the walls of the intestine. Movement is difficult or impossible. (Ref. 2, p. 377)

15. E. All but penicillin therapy have been associated with persistent jaundice during the first month of life, suggesting a disorder called "inspissated bile syndrome." (Ref. 2, p. 379)

16. D. Direct bilirubin is not elevated. There is some evidence to suggest that maternal hormone substances in milk interfere with bilirubin metabolism, but this defect does not involve the excretion of the conjugated form of bilirubin. (Ref. 2, p. 380)

17. C. Trisomy 18 is one of the more frequent chromosomal abnormalities associated with single umbilical artery. (Ref. 2, p. 391)

18. D. Tetany is usually associated with transient hypoparathyroidism and not thyroid deficiency. (Ref. 2, p. 393)

19. E. Newborns with severe illnesses may develop hypoglycemia as a result of increased metabolic needs that are out of proportion to substrate stores. Hyperoxia by itself is not a stimulus for hypoglycemia. (Ref. 2, p. 397)

20. A. Down syndrome, meningomyelocele, and erythroblastosis fetalis can all be diagnosed by amniotic fluid analysis; however, achondroplasia cannot. (Ref. 1, p. 236)

21. B. Duodenal and esophageal atresia are associated with polyhydramnios, whereas renal agenesis and pulmonary hypoplasia are associated with oligohydramnios. (Ref. 2, p. 330)

22. C. The maternal urine estriol levels serve as a good index of placental function and are correlated with fetal size. They cannot be used to estimate gestational age or diagnose preeclampsia. (Ref. 1, p. 112)

23. B. Ultrasound can reliably determine crown rump length and biparietal diameter but is a poor predictor of fetal weight and cannot reliably determine the sex of a fetus. (Ref. 1, p. 110)

24. A. Intrauterine growth retardation is associated with maternal drug addiction, smoking, and malnutrition. Aspirin abuse is associated with neonatal platelet dysfunction but not growth retardation. (Ref. 1, p. 155)

25. B. Multiple births frequently produce infants with a difference in weight of 25% or greater. The mortality among multiple gestations is seven times that of single births. Many twin births can occur vaginally without increased risk, but premature onset of labor is a frequent complication. (Ref. 1, p. 153)

26. **B,C.** Both rectal bleeding and Epstein pearls can be normal
27. **D.** variants. Apt test is used to determine if the blood is
28. **E.** of maternal origin. Horseshoe kidney is one of the
29. **A.** malformations found in trisomy 18. Congenital ne-
30. **E.** phrosis and hydrops fetalis are both associated with
generalized edema, and Turner syndrome is associated with localized edema of the extremities. (Ref. 2, pp. 298,332–333)

31. **D.** Neonatal narcotic addiction can be a serious disease,
32. **E.** and must be suspected when a newborn presents with
33. **E.** the symptoms mentioned, except low birth weight. The
use of drug therapy varies with different hospital centers, and some
institutions have devised scoring systems for determining which
infants should be medicated. Therapy is always indicated if withdrawal is manifested with convulsions. Normally medications are
given for less than two weeks. (Ref. 3, p. 705)

34. **C.** Postmature infants, in addition to showing the signs
35. **E.** mentioned, may often appear more alert than term babies, and are usually below the 50th percentile for weight since
they do not have optimal growth during the additional time they
are in the womb. They require careful observation in the nursery
because of the increased incidence of complications. (Ref. 3,
p. 685)

2 Genetics

DIRECTIONS: Each of the questions or incomplete statements below is followed by five suggested answers or completions. Select the **one** that is best in each case.

---

36. In autosomal dominant inheritance the trait will be found in one parent and
    - A. 25% of daughters and 75% of sons
    - B. 25% of sons and 75% of daughters
    - C. 50% of daughters and 50% of sons
    - D. only in daughters
    - E. none of the above

37. Which of the following statements is NOT correct regarding X-linked inheritance?
    - A. Traits determined by genes carried on the X chromosome may be either recessive or dominant in the female
    - B. Traits determined by genes carried on the X chromosome may be either recessive or dominant in the male
    - C. A female may be heterozygous for an X-linked gene
    - D. Recessive X-linked disorders are occasionally found in females who are homozygous for the disorder
    - E. Males and females have X chromosomes

15

38. 46, XY, 18q- describes a
    A. male with deletion from the long arm of chromosome 18
    B. male with translocation from chromosome 18 to the Y chromosome
    C. male with Klinefelter syndrome
    D. male with trisomy 18 syndrome
    E. normal male karyotype

39. Turner syndrome (45, X) is usually associated with all of the following EXCEPT
    A. mental retardation
    B. short stature
    C. gonadal dysgenesis
    D. primary amenorrhea
    E. broad chest with widely spaced nipples

40. If a person heterozygous for a recessive trait mates with a person heterozygous for the same recessive trait
    A. all of the children show the pathologic trait
    B. 75% of the offspring show the pathologic trait
    C. 50% of the offspring show the pathologic trait
    D. 25% of the offspring show the pathologic trait
    E. none of the offspring are affected

41. Trisomy 18 (Edward syndrome) is usually associated with all of the following EXCEPT
    A. mental retardation
    B. failure to thrive
    C. macrognathia
    D. low set ears
    E. congenital heart disease

42. All of the following are examples of human congenital defects due to the action of pleiotropic genes EXCEPT
    A. Down syndrome with facial and cardiac anomalies
    B. Marfan syndrome with anomalies of the eye, skeleton, and cardiovascular system
    C. osteogenesis imperfecta with blue sclera and oto-sclerosis
    D. acrocephalosyndactyly with abnormalities of skull and extremities
    E. mutation causing kidney agenesis and skeletal anomalies

43. "Marker chromosomes" are
    A. associated with trisomy states
    B. representative of chromosomal deletions
    C. abnormally large chromosomes that cause lethal states
    D. pathologic states of the X chromosome observed in Turner syndrome
    E. not pathognomonic of pathologic states

DIRECTIONS: Each set of lettered headings below is followed by a list of numbered words or phrases. For each numbered word or phrase select

    A   if the item is associated with **A** only,
    B   if the item is associated with **B** only,
    C   if the item is associated with both **A** and **B**,
    D   if the item is associated with neither **A** nor **B**.

    A. Cri-du-chat syndrome
    B. Down syndrome
    C. Both
    D. Neither

44. Autosomal abnormality

45. Associated with an excess of chromosomal material

46. Can be caused by nondisjunction

47. Sex-linked abnormality

48. Caused by an abnormal chromosome 5

    A. Turner syndrome
    B. Klinefelter syndrome
    C. Both
    D. Neither

49. Associated with an abnormal number of X chromosomes

50. Sexual infantilism in adults

51. Seen in both sexes

52. Severe mental retardation is characteristic

53. Can be diagnosed without a karyotype

    A. Hemophilia A
    B. Sickle cell anemia
    C. Both
    D. Neither

54. Inherited as an autosomal disorder

55. All sons of the affected male will also be affected

56. If one parent is affected, the chance of having an affected child is 50%

57. All daughters of an affected father will be carriers

58. Expression of the disease can skip generations in a family

DIRECTIONS: Each group of questions below consists of five lettered headings, followed by a list of numbered words, phrases or statements. For each numbered word, phrase or statement, select the **one** lettered heading that is most closely associated with it. Each lettered heading may be selected once, more than once, or not at all.

Match the diagnostic procedure with the disease it can help diagnose prenatally

    A. Fetal radiography
    B. alpha-fetoprotein measurement in amniotic fluid
    C. Fetal tissue sampling
    D. Ultrasonography
    E. 17-hydroxyprogesterone measurement in amniotic fluid

59. Hemophilia

60. Neural tube defects

61. Hydrocephalus

62. Adrenogenital syndrome

63. Osteogenesis imperfecta

DIRECTIONS: This section consists of situations, each followed by a series of questions. Study each situation, and select the **one** best answer to each question following it.

CASE 1 (Questions 64–68): An infant is born with features of Down syndrome to a 36-year-old primagravida. Both parents are distressed when you discuss the diagnosis with them after your initial assessment of the infant.

64. All of the following may be features of the infant with Down syndrome EXCEPT
    A. hypotonia
    B. simian crease
    C. prominent malformed ears
    D. protruding tongue
    E. hypoplasia of distal phalanx of fifth finger

65. All of the following congenital malformations have an increased incidence in Down syndrome EXCEPT
    A. congenital heart disease, mainly septal defects
    B. cryptorchidism
    C. congenital cataracts
    D. intestinal atresia
    E. imperforate anus

66. All of the following statements are true concerning Down syndrome EXCEPT
    A. about 5% are due to translocation phenomena
    B. a high correlation exists between increased maternal age and increased incidence
    C. there is an increased incidence among male offspring
    D. the frequency of acute leukemia is higher than in the general population
    E. some degree of mental retardation is always found

67. The risk of recurrence for this couple, assuming they both have normal chromosomes, is
    A. 1/200
    B. 1/1000
    C. not completely known
    D. the same as that for another mother who is over the age of 35 years
    E. dependent on family history

68. A recommendation for the care of the infant includes which one of the following?
    A. Genetic counseling for the family
    B. Referral to a neurologist
    C. Immediate institutionalization
    D. Evaluation by a pediatric cardiologist
    E. An IVP to search for kidney malformations

Genetics
Answers and Comments

36. C. Autosomal dominant inheritance indicates that the trait is not sex linked. In a mating in which a parent passes either a normal or a mutant gene to the offspring and the corresponding genes derived from the other parent are normal, 50% of the children will be normal and 50% (male or female) will exhibit the trait. (Ref. 1, p. 232)

37. B. In the male, who has only one X chromosome, a trait will always be expressed. A female can be heterozygous or homozygous for an X-linked gene, but the male can only be homozygous. An X-linked recessive gene in the female is always clinically manifested in the male. (Ref. 1, p. 233)

38. A. Forty-six designates the normal number of chromosomes and XY indicates a male. The designation 18q- pertains to the deletion from the long arm of chromosome 18. (Ref. 1, p. 240)

39. A. Mental retardation is *not* a characteristic feature of Turner syndrome (unlike the other syndromes associated with abnormalities of chromosome number). Mental retardation appears in less than 10% of patients with Turner syndrome. Academic underachievement may be associated with the visual motor perceptual problems found in patients with Turner syndrome. (Ref. 1, p. 1550)

Figure 2

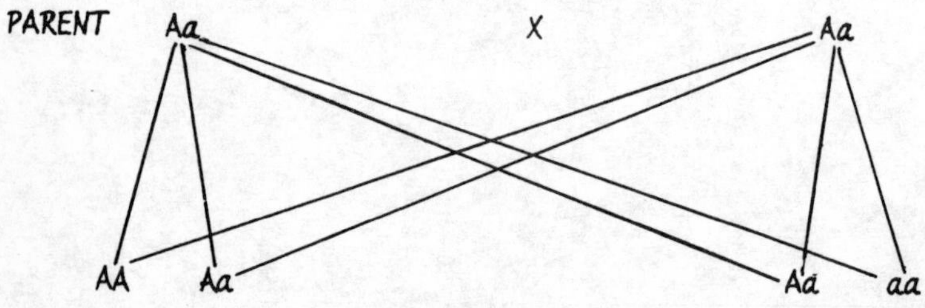

40. D. Twenty-five percent of offspring are affected, i.e., each child has one chance in four of being homozygous and having the pathologic trait (Fig. 2). (Ref. 2, p. 285)

41. C. Micrognathia is associated with trisomy 18 syndrome. The micrognathia has been termed "fish mouth" by some investigators. (Ref. 1, p. 245)

42. A. The anomalies associated with Down syndrome are NOT the result of a pleiotropic effect of a gene mutation but rather of a chromosomal abnormality (trisomy 21). (Ref. 1, p. 231)

43. E. "Marker chromosomes" are normal morphologic variants found in normal karyotypes, e.g., elongation of the centromere region of chromosome numbers 1, 9 and 16. They do not represent pathologic states. (Ref. 2, p. 289)

44. C. Both Down syndrome and cri-du-chat syndrome are au-
45. B. tosomal abnormalities. Down syndrome has an excess
46. A. of genetic material while cri-du-chat has a deletion of
47. D. the short arm of chromosome 5. Neither syndrome is
48. A. sex linked. (Ref. 2, p. 293)

49. C. Turner and Klinefelter syndromes are disorders caused
50. A. by the presence of an abnormal number of X chromo-
51. D. somes (Turner—too few, Klinefelter—too many).
52. D. Turner patients have the female phenotype and are sex-
53. D. ually infantile adults, while those with Klinefelter syndrome are males who develop secondary sex characteristics. Although buccal smears can suggest the diagnosis, a karyotype is mandatory. Severe mental retardation is not seen in either condition. (Ref. 1, pp. 1550, 1553)

54. B. Sickle cell anemia and hemophilia A are recessive dis-
55. D. eases, the expression of which can skip generations. The
56. A. daughters of a father with the sex-linked recessive dis-
57. A. order will all be carriers, and one-half of his children
58. C. (males) will have the disease. Sickle cell disease is an autosomal disorder, and the sex of offspring does not affect inheritance. (Ref. 1, p. 232)

59.	C.	Hemoglobinopathies and hemophilia can now be diag-
60.	B.	nosed prenatally by fetal tissue sampling. An elevated
61.	D.	level of alpha-fetoprotein in amniotic fluid is suggestive
62.	E.	of a neural tube defect, and elevated 17-hydroxypro-
63.	A.	gesterone suggestive of 21 hydroxylase deficiency, a

form of adrenogenital syndrome. Hydrocephalus can be detected by ultrasound, which can also detect valvular heart disease, cystic kidneys and GI obstruction. Fetal radiography can demonstrate poor bone mineralization in a fetus at risk for osteogenesis imperfecta. (Ref. 3, p. 766)

64.	E.	The case presented is that of an infant with Down syn-
65.	C.	drome, and the questions are designed to test basic
66.	C.	knowledge about the syndrome. All of the features
67.	C.	listed, except E, are commonly found, and all of the
68.	A.	malformations mentioned, except C, have an increased

incidence. Hypoplasia of the middle phalanx of the fifth finger may be common, and the incidence of strabismus is also increased. There is no increased male/female ratio in Down syndrome. The risk of recurrence for this couple is not exactly known, but it is increased. There is increasing evidence that paternal nondisjunctions may play a role in this disorder in a significant number of cases. Care of the infant includes proper genetic counseling and enrollment in an infant stimulation program. Immediate institutionalization is no longer recommended (as it frequently was 20 years ago), and there is no need for a neurological or cardiac consultation or IVP routinely. (Ref. 2, p. 298)

3 Developmental and Behavioral Pediatrics

DIRECTIONS: Each of the questions or incomplete statements below is followed by five suggested answers or completions. Select the **one** that is best in each case.

---

69. All of the following are characteristic of psychogenic vomiting EXCEPT
    A. it is usually not seen until after six years of age
    B. it is not associated with food hypersensitivity
    C. in a school age child it may be associated with school phobia
    D. it can be confused with vomiting due to expanding intracranial lesions
    E. it may require psychotherapy

70. Head banging
    A. usually occurs in children three to five years of age
    B. usually occurs in midafternoon
    C. is always associated with mental retardation
    D. is best treated with diazepam
    E. usually requires no major therapeutic intervention

25

71. Mutism in a three-year-old is most likely caused by
   A. congenital or early acquired deafness
   B. mental retardation
   C. hysteria
   D. negativism
   E. severe chorea

72. The most universal cause of growth retardation is
   A. hypoxia secondary to congenital heart disease
   B. malnutrition
   C. repeated respiratory infections
   D. maternal deprivation
   E. chromosomal abnormalities

In caring for adolescents, it is important to understand their normal developmental patterns. The following table is modified from Tanner.

Table 1 Stages of Pubic Hair and Pubertal Genital Development in Males

Stage	Characteristics
1	No pubic hair
2	A little soft thin hair; testes enlarging
3	Some darker curlier hair; skin over testicles thinner; testicles larger
4	More dark, thick, curly hair but not on upper legs; testes getting larger
5	Upper line of hair is straight across and hair now has spread to upper legs

73. During the process of normal adolescent growth and development (Table 1), male gynecomastia is associated with all of the following EXCEPT
   A. it occurs at midpuberty in about 50% of boys
   B. it is usually a transient phenomenon
   C. it usually resolves spontaneously within 18 months
   D. it is usually effectively treated with corticosteroids
   E. it may be of significant psychological concern

74. The first sign of puberty in a normal male is usually the
   A. increase in size of the testes
   B. appearance of facial hair
   C. appearance of auxiliary hair
   D. appearance of pubic hair
   E. appearance of body hair

75. Radiographic examination to determine skeletal maturity is best evaluated by x-rays of the
   A. elbow joint
   B. wrist
   C. ankle
   D. knee joint
   E. hip

76. You are asked to evaluate the developmental status of a one-year-old child. The infant cannot sit without support. He can grasp with one hand, say "baba" and "dada" and respond to "no." He cannot understand the names of objects and does not show interest in pictures. The infant does not creep, cannot stand holding on, and cannot use finger thumb apposition to pick up small objects. He can transfer objects from hand to hand. These observations suggest the infant is
   A. mentally retarded, profound level
   B. mentally retarded, severe-moderate level
   C. functioning at a six to eight month level
   D. functioning at an 11 month level
   E. functioning at age level

77. A seven-year-old child has had no problems until he begins school and has to repeat the first grade. No diagnostic evaluation has been performed. The diagnosis may be any of the following EXCEPT
   A. mild mental retardation
   B. unrecognized seizure state
   C. progressive degenerate neurologic disease
   D. problem is of no concern; the child is a "late bloomer"
   E. previously undetected organic handicap such as hearing loss

78. Which of the following is pathognomonic of attentional deficit disorder?
   A. Soft neurologic signs
   B. Characteristic EEG changes
   C. Psychological evaluation
   D. Type of specific learning disabilities
   E. None of the above

79. A four-year-old is suspected of being mentally retarded. Which of the following would be useful in determining the child's IQ?
   A. Boehm Test of Basic Concepts
   B. Denver Developmental Screening Test
   C. Meeting Street School Screening Test
   D. Gesell Developmental Scales
   E. None of the above

80. Which of the following comments does NOT apply to the Stanford–Binet Intelligence Scale?
   A. Can be used from age two years to adult
   B. Yields a mental age and intelligence quotient
   C. Can correlate with school achievement
   D. Some elements of cultural bias
   E. An exam heavily weighted with visual items

81. Which of the following examinations has a high predictive value in identifying a preschooler with specific learning disabilities?
   A. Denver Developmental Screening Test
   B. Thematic Apperception Test
   C. Peabody Picture Vocabulary Test
   D. Stanford–Binet Intelligence Scales
   E. None of the above

82. Breath holding is characterized by all of the following EXCEPT
   A. it may be similar to a temper tantrum
   B. it may be seen in young infants when startled
   C. in severe cases there may be a momentary lapse of consciousness
   D. symptoms may result from hypoxia
   E. at the height of the attack, the child should be disciplined

---

DIRECTIONS: Each group of questions below consists of five lettered headings, followed by a list of numbered words, phrases or statements. For each numbered word, phrase or statement, select the **one** lettered heading that is most closely associated with it. Each lettered heading may be selected once, more than once, or not at all.

   A. Four month old
   B. Fifteen month old
   C. Three-year-old
   D. Five-year-old
   E. None of the above

83. All deciduous teeth present

84. Stuttering may be normal

85. Babinski reflex normally present

86. Knows own age and sex

87. Can skip

DIRECTIONS: This section consists of situations, each followed by a series of questions. Study each situation, and select the **one** best answer to each question following it.

CASE 1 (Questions 88–90): During a routine check up at 3 weeks of age, you note that the infant appears fussy, and the mother fatigued. Your questioning of the parents suggests a diagnosis of infantile colic.

88. True statements concerning this condition include all of the following EXCEPT
    A. onset is usually in the first few weeks of life
    B. course is self-limited and the prognosis is excellent
    C. recurrence in future infants seems to be unpredictable, though less common than with a first baby
    D. the exact cause is unknown
    E. it does not occur in breastfed infants

89. Actions that may help to decrease symptoms include each of the following EXCEPT
    A. avoidance of excessive stimulation
    B. smaller more frequent feedings
    C. rhythmic rocking
    D. wrapping the infant snugly in a blanket with firm holding
    E. elimination of suspect foods from a breastfeeding mother's diet

90. Medications that have been used for this condition with varying success include all of the following EXCEPT
    A. phenobarbital
    B. whiskey
    C. antihistamines
    D. Bentyl syrup
    E. Lomotil

CASE 2 (Questions 91–92): A mother brings her five-year-old boy to you because he has occasional episodes of wetting the bed at night.

91. True statements about this disorder include each of the following EXCEPT
   A. most children demonstrate other significant psychiatric disturbances
   B. the onset of primary enuresis is before age five years
   C. there is frequently a positive family history
   D. there is no associated urinary tract pathology in most cases
   E. an IVP is not routinely indicated in the work-up

92. Treatment modalities for this condition include all of the following EXCEPT
   A. restriction of fluid intake at night
   B. use of buzzer and pad
   C. use of imipramine
   D. deferring micturition during the day (daytime training)
   E. the use of tolnaftate

Developmental and Behavioral Pediatrics Answers and Comments

69. A. Psychogenic vomiting can occur at any age. It may be a symptom of emotional maladjustment or a serious neurotic disorder. (Ref. 1, p. 920)

70. E. Head banging occurs in perfectly normal children. It is seen usually between six and 12 months of age, occurs usually at bedtime and, for the most part, runs a benign course and stops without therapy. (Ref. 1, p. 75)

71. A. Mutism is usually related to deafness. The other causes listed are possible but are not as common as deafness, which must always be considered in any form of language disorder. (Ref. 1, p. 69)

72. B. Malnutrition is the most universal cause of growth retardation. Depending on the type of malnutrition, growth can be retarded either by diminished cell size or as a result of decreased cell multiplication. (Ref. 1, p. 201)

73. D. All of the other statements regarding male gynecomastia in adolescence are correct. The gynecomastia is usually of great concern to the male adolescent and counseling is necessary to stress the transient nature of the phenomenon. Steroids are not recommended. (Ref. 2, p. 1501)

74. A. The appearance of pubic hair growth usually follows the increase in size of the testes, which coincides with the onset of the adolescent growth (height) spurt. Facial, body, and axillary hair usually appear approximately two years after the growth of pubic hair. (Ref. 1, p. 92)

75. B. The hand and the wrist are the preferred sites for several reasons: (1) convenience, (2) variety and number of developing bones present, and (3) the information documented about this area. (Ref. 1, p. 199)

76. C. The milestones that this child has achieved correspond to those of an infant six to eight months of age. At one year, he should be able to stand holding on, walk with support, say two to three words with meaning, and understand names of objects. The label "mental retardation" cannot be applied until more data are available; for example, can the child see and hear? Although delays in multiple areas suggest mental retardation the infant requires more extensive diagnostic evaluation. In essence, a level of functional ability is designated but more data are required before classification is attempted. (Ref. 2, p. 36)

77. D. The child may have any one of the disorders listed. To the list could be added: attentional deficit disorder, specific learning disabilities, or previously undetected vision and hearing loss. The diagnosis of "late bloomer" or maturational lag, without investigation of other possibilities, is not recommended. (Ref. 1, p. 1576)

78. E. There are no pathognomonic signs of attentional deficit disorder. The diagnosis is based on cumulative data from history and physical and psychological evaluation. The disorder may be suggested by the complex of symptoms: hyperactivity, short attention span, impulsivity, distractibility, and school failure despite average intelligence. (Ref. 1, p. 1616)

79. E. None of the screening tests listed are of value in I.Q. determinations. They are all screening tests and should not be used to assess an intelligence quotient. Probably the best test to use for a four-year-old would be the Stanford–Binet Intelligence Scale or the Wechsler Preschool and Primary Scale of Infant Intelligence. (Ref. 1, pp. 24, 25, 61)

80. E. By about age six this examination is verbally oriented and it may penalize the child with learning problems. The examination is not grouped into verbal and performance subtests. (Ref. 1, pp. 24, 25, 61)

81. E. At the present time there is no single examination, or test battery, that has good predictive value for detecting the preschooler who will have difficulty in school. General intelligence can be assessed, but identification of specific learning disabilities cannot. Perceptual norms for preschoolers have not been well defined. (Ref. 1, pp. 24, 25)

82. E. The child cannot be disciplined during the attack because he has a temporary loss of objectivity. Punishment is not effective in handling breath holding. Ignoring the behavior can reduce its incidence when it is used as a tantrum. (Ref. 2, p. 20)

83. C,D. The primary teeth normally are erupted by age two
84. B,C. years, and the permanent teeth begin to erupt at age
85. A. six. Stuttering may be normal until age four. The Ba-
86. C,D. binski reflex normally may be present until one year
87. D. of age. A five-year-old is expected to skip, know colors, and can dress and undress. A three-year-old is expected to ride a tricycle, and knows age and sex. (Ref. 2, pp. 42, 138, 1020)

88. E. All of the statements, except E, are true concerning
89. B. colic. The most important aspect of treatment is proper
90. E. counseling of the parents, with reassurance that the condition is self-limited. Smaller and more frequent feeding is the only therapy mentioned that does not help the situation. All of the drugs mentioned, except E, have been tried, but at present there is no single drug therapy that works in all affected infants. (Ref. 3, p. 760)

91. A. Enuresis is essentially a benign disorder that often is
92. E. familial and affects mostly boys. Most children with enuresis are well adjusted and healthy. There is an incidence of urinary tract infections in affected children, but there is no associated structural pathology, hence, an IVP is NOT part of the routine work-up. All of the treatments mentioned, except E, have their advocates, and individual practitioners usually decide what they feel most comfortable using. (Ref. 3, p. 18)

4 Accidents, Poisonings, and Environmental Hazards

DIRECTIONS: Each of the questions or incomplete statements below is followed by five suggested answers or completions. Select the **one** that is best in each case.

---

93. Which of the following statements regarding childhood accidents is FALSE?
    A. The majority of injuries in children of all age groups are sustained in the home
    B. From birth to 14 years of age, motor vehicle accidents rank first among fatal accidents
    C. Among children one through four years, deaths are primarily caused by fire, burns, and explosions
    D. Accidents occur more frequently among boys than girls
    E. Some children are accident prone, and accidents cannot be prevented in this group

35

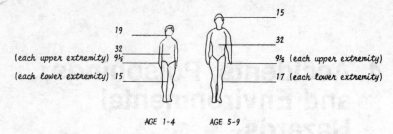

Figure 3 In caring for children with burns, it is important to accurately assess the extent of the burn. Charts such as these are helpful. The numbers represent percentage of body burns.

94. The most common cause of burns in children (Fig. 3) is related to
    A. low-voltage household current
    B. flammable clothing
    C. scalding by spilling or immersion
    D. chemically strong acids
    E. contact with high-voltage wires

95. Which of the following statements is true of a second-degree burn of the leg in a five-year-old child?
    A. The use of hexachlorophene as a cleansing agent is contraindicated
    B. Routinely, the burned area is covered with a topical antibiotic
    C. The child should be given hyperimmune human anti-tetanus serum
    D. Routine administration of an oral broad spectrum antibiotic is recommended
    E. Immediate hospitalization is required

96. A child with gastroenteritis, stupor, convulsions, and circulatory collapse was reported to have ingested something from a plant. The most suspicious plant would be
    A. seeds of larkspur
    B. flowers of oleander
    C. seeds of jimsonweed
    D. castor beans and seeds
    E. leaves of azalea

97. Gastric lavage is contraindicated after ingestion of
    A. aspirin
    B. corrosive alkali
    C. diazepam
    D. castor beans
    E. vitamins

98. A four-year-old has confirmed salicylate toxicity. The first sign is usually
    A. petechiae and gingival bleeding
    B. diplopia and peripheral blindness
    C. hyperventilation
    D. diarrhea and vomiting
    E. convulsions

99. A two-year-old child has ingested toxic amounts of iron (as an oral hematinic). The first sign to be noted within the first hour is
    A. vomiting and bloody diarrhea
    B. tremors, convulsions, and coma
    C. hyperventilation
    D. petechiae and bleeding from the gums
    E. hallucinations

100. The toxicity of petroleum distillates is related to
    A. aspiration of hydrocarbon into the respiratory tract
    B. gastric ulceration and hemorrhage
    C. CNS depression, convulsions, and coma
    D. renal parenchyma destruction and renal failure
    E. hemolysis of red blood cells and hemoglobinuria

101. An adolescent presents to an emergency room in coma, with constricted pupils, respiratory depression, cyanosis, and rales. The most likely diagnosis is
    A. bilateral bronchopneumonia
    B. acute heroin toxicity
    C. acute amphetamine toxicity
    D. an LSD trip
    E. too much whiskey

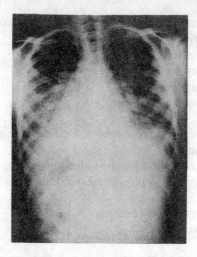

Figure 4 An example of the chest of a person who almost drowned.

102. The most commonly abused pharmacologic agent(s) is
    A. marijuana and barbiturates
    B. cocaine
    C. LSD
    D. heroin
    E. alcohol

103. In approximately what percentage of drowning victims is aspiration (Fig. 4) NOT a cause of death?
    A. 50%
    B. 10%
    C. 75%
    D. 2%
    E. 0.5%

DIRECTIONS: Each group of questions below consists of lettered headings, followed by a list of numbered words, phrases, or statements. For **each** numbered word, phrase, or statement select the **one** lettered heading that is most closely associated with it. Each lettered heading may be selected once, more than once, or not at all.

Questions 104–108 Many drugs are useful in treating acute intoxications in children. Match the drug with the corresponding ingestion.

    A. Organophosphate and carbamate insecticides
    B. Iron poisoning
    C. Lye ingestion
    D. Phenothiazine ingestion with extrapyramidal reaction
    E. Ethanol ingestion
    F. Methemoglobinemia
    G. Lead ingestion

104. Prednisone

105. Atropine sulfate

106. Benadryl

107. Deferoxamine

108. D-penicillamine

Accidents, Poisonings, and Environmental Hazards
Answers and Comments

93. **E.** Accident proneness is a controversial issue. It does not eliminate the need for adult supervision of the dangerous environment. Indeed, it demands more adult concern for such a child's surroundings. Virtually all accidents are preventable. The hyperactive, impulsive, short-attentioned, emotionally labile child may be more prone to accidents but needs tighter supervision as a preventive measure. Be sure to check visual acuity in children with recurrent accidents! (Ref. 1, p. 725)

94. **C.** Spilling a hot liquid onto oneself and immersion in scalding liquids represent the most common etiology for burns in childhood. Scald burns are less likely to be fatal than immersion scald burns because of the differences in surface area involved. (Ref. 1, p. 718)

95. **A.** The use of hexachlorophene is contraindicated because surface absorption may result in neurotoxicity. Topical antibiotics are not utilized for outpatient care in some centers. (Others may apply a Silvadine dressing.) Superficial burns such as this are not tetanus prone. Routine antibiotics are not necessary. (Ref. 1, p. 720)

96. **D.** From the list one would think first of castor bean because of the characteristic features described. The poisonous substance of the castor bean is ricin. Larkspur causes CNS excitation; oleander CNS depression, bradyarrhythmia; jimsonweed has an atropinelike effect, and azalea has a curarelike effect. (Ref. 1, p. 746)

97. **B.** Gastric lavage would be indicated for all of the accidental ingestions, except corrosive agents. The risk involves possible perforation of the esophagus. Children with strychnine, glutethimide, barbiturate, or antihistamine poisoning may require prior endotracheal intubation because of the danger of laryngospasm. (Ref. 1, p. 726)

98. C. Toxic levels of salicylate produce an encephalopathy with primary disturbance of the respiratory center of the medulla, resulting in a primary hyperpnea. A result of this is reduced pCO_2, which causes a rise in plasma pH. (Ref. 1, p. 732)

99. A. The first phase of iron toxicity usually begins within 30 to 60 minutes after ingestion. Usually the initial symptoms are vomiting and bloody diarrhea; acidemia and circulatory collapse may develop. (Ref. 1, p. 729)

100. A. Aspiration of hydrocarbon into the respiratory tract causes local irritation, pneumonitis, hemorrhagic bronchopneumonia, atelectasis, and pulmonary edema. Complications include pneumatoceles, effusions, and pneumothorax. Extensive lesions in the lungs can cause death within 24 hours after ingestion. (Ref. 1, p. 737)

101. B. Until proven otherwise, the patient must be considered to have overdosed on heroin. Methadone overdose is identical to that of heroin. Toxicity from barbiturates also resembles that from opiates. (Ref. 1, p. 753)

102. E. Alcohol is still the mostly commonly abused agent. Teenagers use and experiment with alcohol, more so than with tobacco or marijuana. It is estimated that there are 500,000 teenage alcoholics. (Ref. 1, p. 759)

103. B. Ten percent of victims die of laryngospasm or breath holding. With prompt resuscitation, recovery is complete. (Ref. 2, p. 262)

104. C. Prednisone may be useful in reducing scarring after
105. A. ingestion of caustic substances such as lye. Atropine is
106. D. often used in treating intoxication with organophosphate
107. B. insecticides because it antagonizes the parasympathetic
108. G. effects of these compounds. Pralidoxime is also given concurrently in more severe cases. Benadryl is the treatment of choice and can have dramatic results for tardive dyskinesia-type reactions to phenothiazines. Deferoxamine and penicillamine are used for iron and lead poisonings, respectively. (Ref. 3, p. 654)

5 Nutrition

DIRECTIONS: Each of the questions or incomplete statements below is followed by five suggested answers or completions. Select the **one** that is best in each case.

---

109. Amino acids in excess of needs for protein synthesis and other nitrogen compounds are handled in all of the following ways EXCEPT
    A. excreted as ammonia
    B. stored as amino acids in the liver
    C. synthesized into energy yielding compounds
    D. synthesized into storage compounds such as fat
    E. excreted as urea

110. Essential amino acids for the neonate which are the same as for the older child include all of the following EXCEPT
    A. valine
    B. lysine
    C. leucine
    D. phenylalanine
    E. cystine

111. In comparing the lipid content of human milk with that of modified cow milk formula, all of the following are true EXCEPT
    A. the cholesterol content of human milk is highest
    B. the lipid composition of human milk contains more saturated fatty acids
    C. human milk is higher in essential fatty acids
    D. avoidance of human milk for infant feeding is a proven preventative measure for atheromatous disease in later life if there is a family history of hyperlipidemia
    E. human milk is easily absorbed by the infant

112. Patients at risk for pernicious anemia include all of the following EXCEPT
    A. vegetarians who include milk and eggs in their diet
    B. postgastrectomy patients
    C. patients with ileal resection
    D. patients lacking intrinsic factor for B_{12} absorption
    E. vegetarians who consume large amounts of nut proteins

113. Colostrum has all of the following properties EXCEPT
    A. it has a higher fat content than mature milk
    B. it has a higher protein content than mature milk
    C. it is richer in vitamin A, compared with mature human milk
    D. sodium and potassium are higher than in mature human milk
    E. it contains protective antibodies

Breastfeeding may be contraindicated if the mother *must* take certain drugs regularly, which are themselves contraindicated. This table lists the most important ones.

Table 2 Drugs Contraindicated in the Breastfeeding Mother

All anticancer agents

All antithyroid medications

Any medicine containing atropine

Oral contraceptives

Laxatives that are anthraquinone derivatives (cascara, senna)

Lithium

Corticosteroids in high doses

Antibiotics: INH,* Flagyl, chloramphenicol, tetracyclines, sulfonamides (certain situations), griseofulvin

Antihypertensives: reserpine, Hygroton; Diuril (*Physicians Desk Reference* recommendation)

Anticoagulants: phenindione

All narcotics, especially Darvon, methadone, heroin; codeine and morphine seem to be okay

Radioactive pharmaceuticals: gallium, iodine

Nursing should cease for 48 hours after use of technetium

Note:
All drugs should be used with caution.

Observe for physical or behavioral changes in the infant.

Always check for information in the *Physicians Desk Reference*.

Contact your local poison control center if in doubt about a given drug.

*Potential risks must be weighed against benefits in certain populations.

(Adapted from LaCerva: *Breastfeeding: A Manual for Health Professionals*.)

114. An absolute contraindication to breastfeeding (Table 2) is
   A. erythroblastosis fetalis
   B. inverted nipples
   C. mastitis
   D. cigarette smoking
   E. active tuberculosis in the mother

115. All of the following apply to a comparison between breast milk and cow's milk EXCEPT
    A. breast milk produces a lower stool pH
    B. breast milk produces higher counts of lactobacillus in stools
    C. breast milk produces high concentrations of secretory IgA
    D. breast milk has a lower caloric content
    E. fat absorption by infant is better with breast milk

116. All of the following observations might be indicators of the adequacy of breast milk supply EXCEPT
    A. if the infant appears satisfied
    B. if the infant sleeps two to four hours between feedings
    C. if the infant exhibits adequate weight gain
    D. if the mother has a let down reflex and feels breasts are emptied after feedings
    E. if the infant rarely cries

117. Concerning colostrum, which of the following statements is FALSE?
    A. It has an alkaline reaction
    B. 10 to 40 ml daily are secreted
    C. It contains less protein than breast milk that is more mature
    D. It contains less carbohydrate and fat than mature breast milk
    E. It contains maternal leukocytes

118. Vitamin A deficiency can be expected to occur with all of the following EXCEPT
    A. chronic ingestion of mineral oil
    B. a low-fat diet
    C. pancreatic disease
    D. celiac disease
    E. a lack of yellow vegetables in the diet

119. Hypervitaminosis A may be associated with all of the following EXCEPT
    A. acute ingestion of 300,000 IU of vitamin A
    B. symptoms of pseudotumor cerebri
    C. anorexia and vomiting
    D. blood levels of retinol in the range of 20 to 50μg/dl
    E. desquamation of the skin

120. The breastfed infant of a mother with severe beriberi would be expected to exhibit all of the following EXCEPT
    A. restlessness, anorexia, vomiting, and constipation
    B. undernourishment
    C. rapid heart rate and enlarged liver
    D. edema restricted to the head and trunk
    E. waxy skin

121. Niacin deficiency is characterized by
    A. an increased incidence in patients on vegetarian diets with milk and eggs included
    B. diarrhea, dermatitis, and dementia
    C. a dermatitis that responds to exposure to sunlight
    D. a decreased incidence in fall and winter
    E. high morbidity

122. Pyridoxine deficiency may be associated with all of the following EXCEPT
    A. seizure disorder
    B. isoniazid ingestion
    C. a macrocytic anemia
    D. ingestion of prolonged heat-processed formula by infants
    E. inherited inability to utilize normal amounts of pyridoxine

123. The need for vitamin C is increased by all of the following EXCEPT
    A. infectious disease
    B. iron deficiency
    C. smoking
    D. cold exposure
    E. protein excess in the diet

124. Defects in the formation of which of the following explain most of the clinical findings in scurvy?
A. Phospholipid
B. Protein
C. Endothelium
D. Glycogen
E. Collagen

125. Scurvy is a manifestation of a deficiency of which of the following?
A. Vitamin C
B. Vitamin B
C. Vitamin K
D. Vitamin E
E. Vitamin A

126. A ten-month-old infant with known iron deficiency, fed solely on cow's milk, develops painful lower extremities, refuses to walk, and assumes a frog leg position when resting. The most likely nutritional disorder is
A. protein calorie malnutrition
B. vitamin D rickets
C. scurvy
D. B complex deficiency
E. vitamin A deficiency

127. The diagnosis of scurvy is usually made by
A. blood assay
B. tissue biopsy
C. x-ray of long bones
D. assay of nail content
E. radioactive isotope methods

128. The vitamin deficiency that produces osteomalacia in non-growing bone is
A. vitamin C
B. vitamin A
C. vitamin B_6
D. vitamin B_2
E. vitamin D

129. Which of the following statements concerning vitamin D metabolism is FALSE?
    A. Bound to alpha-2 globulin in lymphatics
    B. Requires bile for absorption
    C. Kidney is active in metabolism
    D. Circulates in plasma as 25-OH cholecalciferol
    E. Stored in the liver but not metabolized there

130. In the absence of vitamin D, serum calcium may be maintained by
    A. parathyroid hormone secretion
    B. decreased renal excretion of phosphate
    C. small dietary increases
    D. decreased renal excretion of alkali
    E. increased amounts of vitamin A in the diet

131. Clinical disorders associated with increased incidence of vitamin D deficiency include all of the following EXCEPT
    A. cystic fibrosis
    B. hepatic disease
    C. celiac disease
    D. renal disease
    E. obesity

132. All of the following are effects of parathyroid hormone EXCEPT
    A. hypophosphatemia
    B. hyperphosphaturia
    C. calcium release from bone
    D. reduced renal clearance of calcium
    E. decreased calcium absorption from the gut

133. Which of the following statements concerning calcitonin is FALSE?
    A. It is secreted by the kidney
    B. It inhibits bone resorption
    C. It lowers serum calcium in hypercalcemia
    D. The activity of calcitonin increases with increasing levels of serum phosphate
    E. A thyroidectomy causes decreased secretion of calcitonin

134. All of the following are clinical signs of rickets EXCEPT
    A. craniotabes
    B. enlargement of the costochondral junctions
    C. thickening of wrists and ankles
    D. poor growth
    E. conjunctivitis

135. The daily requirement for vitamin D is.
    A. 100 IU
    B. 400 IU
    C. 600 IU
    D. 1000 IU
    E. 50 IU

136. Rickets may be treated by all of the following EXCEPT
    A. sunlight
    B. 1500 to 5000 IU of vitamin D daily for two to four weeks
    C. 600,000 IU of vitamin D as a single dose
    D. sunlight plus 1500 to 5000 IU of vitamin D daily until healing is demonstrated on x-ray
    E. increased calcium in the diet, and decreased phosphate

137. Symptoms of hypervitaminosis D include all of the following EXCEPT
    A. hypotonia
    B. polydipsia and polyuria
    C. irritability
    D. hypocalcemia
    E. metastatic calcifications

138. Vitamin E deficiency may develop with all of the following EXCEPT
    A. prematures
    B. cystic fibrosis
    C. kwashiorkor
    D. dietary intake of 1 mg of vitamin E per 0.6 g of unsaturated fat in the diet
    E. biliary atresia

139. Which of the following statements concerning body water is FALSE?
    A. TBW decreases from 78% of body weight at birth to 60% at one year of age
    B. Extracellular fluid volume is larger than intracellular space in the fetus
    C. Extracellular fluid volume is approximately 40% of body weight in the older child
    D. Intracellular fluid volume is approximately 30 to 40% of body weight
    E. TBW (liters) = 0.611 wt (kg) $\pm$ 0.251

140. The principal regulatory mechanism for water excretion is
    A. glomerular filtration rate
    B. the adrenal gland
    C. antidiuretic hormone
    D. the state of the renal tubular epithelium
    E. the sweat gland

141. Total body sodium is depleted in all of the following EXCEPT
    A. hyponatremic dehydration
    B. isonatremic dehydration
    C. hypernatremic dehydration
    D. Addison disease
    E. Cushing disease

142. Which is the appropriate IV fluid for initial hydration of the patient with severe hypernatremic dehydration?
    A. Five percent glucose in water
    B. Isotonic saline with potassium
    C. Ten percent glucose in water
    D. Sodium in glucose solution without potassium
    E. Two and one-half percent glucose in water

143. Improvement in a hospitalized infant who had failed to gain weight and was developmentally slow at home would suggest
    A. an infectious etiology
    B. carbon monoxide poisoning
    C. psychosocial factors
    D. rumination syndrome
    E. food intolerance

DIRECTIONS: Each set of lettered headings below is followed by a list of numbered words or phrases. For each numbered word or phrase select

A   if the item is associated with **A** only,
B   if the item is associated with **B** only,
C   if the item is associated with both **A** and **B**,
D   if the item is associated with neither **A** nor **B**.

A. Breast milk
B. Cow's milk
C. Both
D. Neither

144. Greater protein concentration

145. Approximately 24 cal/oz

146. 80% casein, 20% whey protein

147. Greater lactose concentration

148. Calcium/phosphorus ratio of about 2:1

DIRECTIONS: Each group of questions below consists of lettered headings, followed by a list of numbered words, phrases, or statements. For each numbered word, phrase, or statement, select the **one** lettered heading that is most closely associated with it. Each lettered heading may be selected once, more than once, or not at all.

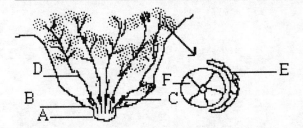

Figure 5 Labels in diagram of a normal breast to be used in answering Questions 149–153.

149. Via stimulation of oxytocin, produces let-down

150. Via stimulation of prolactin, produces breastmilk

151. Trauma or blockage produces segmental engorgement

152. Stimulation results in an increase of prolactin

153. Specialized lubricating glands

    A. Vitamin A
    B. Vitamin B$_6$
    C. Vitamin C
    D. Vitamin D
    E. Vitamin E

154. Deficiency causes peripheral neuropathy

155. Deficiency causes bleeding problems

156. Deficiency may be a problem in some breastfed infants

157. Deficiency causes night blindness

158. Deficiency more common in low birth-weight infants

Nutrition
Answers and Comments

109. B. There is no storage facility for amino acids. (Ref. 1, p. 182)

110. E. Fetuses, small premature infants, and possibly some full-term infants may have a very limited capacity to convert methionine to cysteine and cystine. (Ref. 1, p. 182)

111. D. Avoidance of higher cholesterol content of human milk has not been proved to modify atheromatous disease of later life. It is an area under investigation. (Ref. 1, p. 219)

112. A. B_{12} is present in sufficient amounts in egg and milk products and will protect the patient who has excluded meat from his diet. (Ref. 1, p. 216)

113. A. Colostrum has less fat and sugar than mature milk. (Ref. 1, p. 220)

114. E. Active tuberculosis is an absolute contraindication as are other serious maternal infections, especially if they require drugs that are contraindicated when nursing. (Ref. 2, p. 150)

115. D. Total caloric content is the same, but caloric distribution is significantly different. (Ref. 2, pp. 150, 155)

116. E. Infants cry for many reasons other than hunger. Usually the best single indicator of adequate breast milk supply is growth of the infant. (Ref. 2, p. 149)

117. C. Colostrum contains several times as much protein as mature breast milk. (Ref. 2, p. 198)

118. E. All of the choices presented, except the lack of yellow vegetables in the diet, can result in low intake or poor absorption of vitamin A. Fruit, eggs, butter, and liver provide adequate amounts of vitamin A. (Ref. 2, p. 170)

119. D. Blood levels of retinol in the range of 20 to 50 μg/dl are normal for infants. (Ref. 2, p. 172)

120. D. Congenital beriberi has been described in breastfed infants of mothers with severe beriberi. They usually become symptomatic during the first three months of life. The edema, if present, is usually restricted to the distal parts of the extremities. (Ref. 2, p. 173)

121. B. The classic triad of pellagra consists of diarrhea, dermatitis, and dementia. (Ref. 2, p. 174)

122. C. The anemia of pyridoxine deficiency is a microcytic hypochromic anemia associated with failure of iron utilization in hemoglobin synthesis. (Ref. 2, p. 175)

123. E. Protein *depletion* may increase the need for vitamin C. (Ref. 2, p. 176)

124. E. Ascorbate and oxygen are essential for formation of normal collagen. (Ref. 2, p. 176)

125. A. Vitamin C deficiency will result in a symptom complex called scurvy. (Ref. 2, p. 176)

126. C. A diet consisting solely of cow's milk would be deficient in vitamin C. The pain-associated periosteal lesions cause pseudoparalysis. (Ref. 2, p. 176)

127. C. Laboratory tests for scurvy are unsatisfactory. The characteristic clinical picture and history are valuable in diagnosis. (Ref. 2, p. 178)

128. E. Rickets is characterized by formation of normal collagen and matrix and of osteoid, with defective mineralization. (Ref. 2, p. 179)

129. E. Vitamin D is hydroxylated to 25-OH cholecalciferol in the liver. (Ref. 2, p. 179)

130. A. Parathyroid hormone will mobilize calcium from bone. (Ref. 2, p. 180)

131. E. Obesity itself has not been associated with increased incidence of vitamin D deficiency. (Ref. 2, p. 179)

132. E. Parathyroid hormone causes increased calcium absorption from the intestine, and this action is enhanced by 1,25 hydroxycholecalciferol. (Ref. 2, p. 180)

133. A. Calcitonin is secreted by the thyroid. (Ref. 2, p. 180)

134. E. All of the choices given except conjunctivitis are fairly early signs of rickets that occur after several months of vitamin D deficiency. (Ref. 2, p. 181)

135. B. This amount is present in either 32 oz of whole milk or a 13 oz can of evaporated milk. (Ref. 2, p. 179)

136. E. While it may be helpful and advisable in some cases to correct disturbances in Ca/P ratios in the diet, this alone will not be useful in the treatment of rickets. (Ref. 2, p. 183)

137. D. Hypercalcemia and hypercalciuria are notable. Differential diagnosis includes chronic nephritis, hyperparathyroidism, and idiopathic hypercalcemia. (Ref. 2, p. 184)

138. D. Prematures have poor absorption of vitamin E and patients with malabsorption are at risk. The minimum daily requirement of vitamin E is not known but 1 mg per 0.6 g of unsaturated fat in the diet appears adequate. Premature infants should receive at least 5 mg daily. (Ref. 2, p. 184)

139. C. Extracellular fluid volume is approximately 20% of body weight. (Ref. 2, p. 206)

140. C. Urine volume is influenced by diet and can be reduced only to that necessary to excrete solute load. (Ref. 2, p. 208)

141. D. Serum electrolyte values indicate the relative losses of water and electrolytes. Patients with Addison disease will enter negative sodium balance because of inappropriately elevated urine sodium. Cushing disease results in positive sodium balance because of increased steroid production with mineral corticoid effects. (Ref. 2, p. 211)

142. D. Sick infants should be provided with glucose to combat hypoglycemia. Potassium should be given only after renal function has been established. (Ref. 2, p. 236)

143. C. The child's intake of calories is very often substandard because of psychosocial circumstances that are not clear at first glance. Maternal deprivation is the most common cause of failure to thrive in the United States. (Ref. 2, p. 253)

144. B. Cow's milk has a greater protein concentration, and this
145. D. is one reason why breast milk is better for newborns: it
146. B. creates less of a renal solute load. Both cow and breast
147. A. milk have about 20 cal/oz, though this will vary some-
148. A. what with a given sample. The greater concentration of casein in cow's milk is believed to contribute to an increased incidence of constipation. Breast milk is higher in carbohydrate concentration, though the milk sugar (lactose) is the same in both. Breast milk has a more favorable Ca/P ratio which enhances the absorption of calcium from the gut. (Ref. 3, p. 713 and Ref. 2, p. 155)

149. E. The myoepithelial cells contract via oxytocin stimula-
150. F. tion, thus, forcing milk from the milk producing cells
151. D. into the ductular system. Engorgement is produced
152. A. when a major duct system does not drain properly, al-
153. B. lowing both breast milk and surrounding tissue fluid to accumulate. Nipple stimulation results in increased production of prolactin and, thus, of breastmilk. The areola contains Montgomery glands, which provide lubrication during sucking. (Ref. 2, p. 396)

154. B. Peripheral neuropathy is a complication of B_6 deficiency,
155. C. and its prevention is the main reason it is given to older
156. D. children on INH. Lack of vitamin C causes both skin
157. A. and periosteal hemorrhages. Rickets has been reported
158. E. in dark skinned urban breastfeeding infants in the winter, and supplementation may be indicated for some of this high risk group. Night blindness is due to a lack of vitamin A, and is still a major public health problem in some third world countries. Vitamin E deficiency seems to contribute to hemolytic anemia in low birth weight infants, though its relationship to retrolental fibroplasia is still uncertain. (Ref. 3, p. 3)

6 Immunologic Disorders

DIRECTIONS: Each of the questions or incomplete statements below is followed by five suggested answers or completions. Select the **one** that is best in each case.

---

159. Which of the following is NOT associated with IgM?
    A. Normally not found in cord blood of newborns
    B. Produced in part in the spleen
    C. Has the longest biologic half-life of all the major immunoglobulins
    D. Comprises 5% to 10% of the total immunoglobulins under normal circumstances
    E. When elevated, usually represents a response to either intrauterine or neonatal infection

160. On laboratory screening, which of the following usually denotes immunodeficiency?
    A. IgG level less than 200 mg/dl
    B. IgM level of 10 mg/dl
    C. Positive Schick test in a completely immunized patient
    D. Total lymphocyte count at any age of 1200/mm^3
    E. IgA level less than 10 mg/dl

161. Depression of T-cell rosettes, as a quantitative in vitro measure of circulating T lymphocytes, is seen in all of the following EXCEPT
   A. acute and chronic viral infection
   B. malignancy
   C. infectious mononucleosis
   D. autoimmune disease
   E. cellular immunodeficiency disorders

162. Which one of the following is NOT characteristic of disorders following splenectomy?
   A. Increased susceptibility to infection with polysaccharide-containing organisms
   B. Splenectomy in a patient with Wiskott–Aldrich syndrome is uniformly fatal
   C. Presence of an adequate number of opsonins in the form of antibody is an important prognostic factor
   D. Age at splenectomy is not an important consideration
   E. Patients with sickle cell disease have an increased susceptibility to pneumococcal infections

163. Lazy leukocyte syndrome is associated with all of the following EXCEPT
   A. defective phagocytic response to normal chemotactic stimuli
   B. normal number of neutrophils
   C. normal humoral and cellular immunity
   D. recurrent low-grade fever, gingivitis, stomatitis, and otitis media
   E. in vitro leukocyte phagocytosis and bacterial killing are normal

164. Which of the following statements concerning chronic granulomatous disease is FALSE?
  A. Basic defect in WBC is deficient respiratory oxidative metabolic activity
  B. Organisms commonly associated with this disease include streptococci and pneumococci
  C. Polymorphonuclear leukocytes normally phagocytize but are defective in bactericidal function
  D. It is inherited primarily as a sex-linked recessive trait
  E. It is evidence of abnormal function of eosinophils and mononuclear phagocytic cells

DIRECTIONS: Each group of questions below consists of lettered headings, followed by a list of numbered words, phrases, or statements. For each numbered word, phrase, or statement, select the **one** lettered heading that is most closely associated with it. Each lettered heading may be selected once, more than once, or not at all.

  A. Chediak–Higashi syndrome
  B. Ataxia–telangiectasia
  C. Wiskott–Aldrich syndrome
  D. DiGeorge syndrome
  E. Nezelof syndrome

165. Sex-linked recessive

166. Abnormality in granulocyte function

167. Associated with hypocalcemia in the neonatal period

168. Cellular immunodeficiency and normal immunoglobulin levels with specific antibody production absent

169. Autosomal recessive disorder with IgA deficiency

170. Associated with neonatal thrombocytopenia

    A. T cell deficiency
    B. B cell deficiency
    C. Both
    D. Neither

171. Congenital hypogammaglobulinemia

172. DiGeorge syndrome

173. Sturge–Weber syndrome

174. Ataxia–telangiectasia

175. Nezelof syndrome

Immunologic Disorders
Answers and Comments

159. C. IgG has the longest half-life of the major immunoglobulins (25 days). IgM has a half-life of only five days. (Ref. 1, p. 407)

160. C. Normal antibody will neutralize diphtheria toxin, and no reaction will be seen following skin testing with Schick reagent. (Ref. 1, p. 412)

161. C. Elevated levels of T cell rosettes have been described in infectious mononucleosis. (Ref. 1, p. 413)

162. D. Age is a very critical factor to consider; splenectomized infants probably should receive antibiotics prophylactically. (Ref. 1, p. 1108)

163. B. Neutropenia is characteristic of this disorder. (Ref. 1, p. 1092)

164. B. Streptococci and pneumococci contain hydrogen peroxide which supplies the defective WBC with this necessary killing ingredient. Chronic granulomatous disease is often accompanied by bacterial infection caused by *Serratia marcescens* or *Staphylococcus epidermidis*. (Ref. 1, p. 1093)

165. C. Wiskott-Aldrich syndrome is the only sex-linked disor-
166. A. der listed and is associated with neonatal thrombocy-
167. D. topenia. DiGeorge syndrome consists of thymic and
168. E. parathyroid aplasia and can present with neonatal hy-
169. B. pocalcemia. The ataxia telangiectasia syndrome most
170. C. commonly exhibits IgA deficiency and is autosomal recessive. Chediak-Higashi syndrome is also autosomal recessive but has no associated IgA abnormality. It does however have an associated dysmorphology of the granulocytes (giant cytoplasmic granular inclusions). Nezelof syndrome is a primary immunodeficiency disease characterized by varying degrees of cellular immunodeficiency and normal or nearly normal immunoglobulin levels. (Ref. 1, pp. 1093, 418–423)

171. **B.** Congenital hypogammaglobulinemia is characterized by
172. **A.** lack of serum immunoglobulins, and can be treated with
173. **D.** i.m. injections of human immune serum globulin, or i.v.
174. **A.** use of modified immune serum globulin. DiGeorge syn-
175. **C.** drome and Ataxia–telangiectasia both have T-cell deficiencies due to underdeveloped or absent thymus gland. Nezelof syndrome has varying degrees of cellular immunodeficiency, normal immunoglobulin levels, but absent specific antibody production. Sturge–Weber syndrome has no associated immunodeficiency. (Ref. 3, pp. 56, 745–747)

7 Allergy

DIRECTIONS: Each of the questions or incomplete statements below is followed by five suggested answers or completions. Select the **one** that is best in each case.

---

176. Which of the following statements does NOT accurately describe childhood asthma?
    A. The intrinsic form is more common than the extrinsic
    B. It represents the classic form of type I immediate hypersensitivity
    C. IgE antibodies are increased
    D. It is associated with the release of slow reacting substance of anaphylaxis
    E. Between attacks the patient may appear symptomatically well

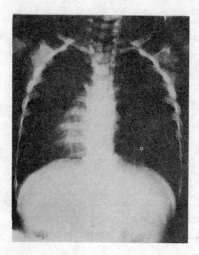 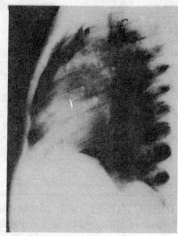

Figure 6 AP (*left*) and lateral (*right*) views of pneumomediastinum in an asthmatic patient.

177. Which of the following is NOT characteristic of asthma (Fig. 6)?
   A. pneumomediastinum may be a complication
   B. aspirin intolerance may be associated
   C. because status asthmaticus does not always involve hypoxemia, it may sometimes be treated at home
   D. theophylline is the drug of choice for patients with moderate asthma who require daily therapy
   E. acute episodes may be precipitated by infection, irritant or allergic exposure, or emotional events

178. Which of the following statements does NOT characterize penicillin allergy?
   A. The metabolic pathway for major determinants is responsible for most anaphylactic reactions
   B. Rash and symptoms like those of serum sickness are caused by IgE antibodies to major pathway products
   C. With large amounts of penicillin, RBC membranes become coated with penicillin G and are recognized as being foreign, and then are lysed
   D. Any of the four types of hypersensitivity response may occur
   E. Blocking antibody can be formed

DIRECTIONS: Each set of lettered headings below is followed by a list of numbered words or phrases. For each numbered word or phrase select

   A   if the item is associated with **A** only,
   B   if the item is associated with **B** only,
   C   if the item is associated with both **A** and **B**,
   D   if the item is associated with neither **A** nor **B**.

   A. Atopic dermatitis
   B. Contact dermatitis
   C. Both
   D. Neither

179. Acute phase manifested by erythema, weeping oozing lesions

180. Burrow's solution useful in acute phase

181. Topical steroids useful to control the disease

182. Frequent bathing helpful

183. Secondary infection with staph or strep is common

DIRECTIONS: Each group of questions below consists of five lettered headings, followed by a list of numbered words, phrases or statements. For each numbered word, phrase or statement, select the **one** lettered heading that is most closely associated with it. Each lettered heading may be selected once, more than once, or not at all.

A. Histamine
B. IgM
C. IgG
D. bradykinin
E. serotonin

184. Produced by hyposensitization, blocking antibody

185. Contributes to anaphylaxis

186. Contributes to urticaria

187. Contributes to angioedema

188. First response to infection

Allergy
Answers and Comments

176. A. Intrinsic asthma is more commonly seen in adults. (Ref. 1, p. 461)

177. C. Status asthmaticus is a serious condition requiring hospital admission, i.v. fluids and medication, and blood gas monitoring. (Ref. 2, p. 544)

178. A. The major penicilloyl determinant causes the formation of IgG antibodies in recently treated patients. These antibodies appear to act as blocking antibodies and prevent IgE mediated anaphylactic reaction. Because large amounts of antigen are required for the formation of IgG antibodies, blocking antibodies to minor determinants do not occur. (Ref. 1, p. 474)

179. C. Atopic dermatitis and contact dermatitis share a number
180. C. of features in common. Their appearance is similar in
181. C. the acute phase, with weeping lesions that respond well
182. D. to the astringent action of an aluminum solution (Bur-
183. C. row's). Both conditions respond well to the administration of topical steroids, and are prone to secondary infection. The main differentiating features are the age of onset, and the distribution. Atopic dermatitis commonly arises in infancy with typical lesions occurring on the cheeks and extensor aspects of the extremities. Contact dermatitis has a distribution related to the irritant involved, and may occur at any age. (Ref. 3, p. 437)

184. B,C. Both IgM and IgG can be blocking antibodies. His-
185. A,D. tamine, bradykinin, and IgE are involved in ana-
186. A. phylaxis. Histamine is the primary mediator for
187. D. urticaria, and bradykinin is for angioedema. The first
188. B. response to an infection is production of IgM, which is followed by IgG. Serotonin has no known role in the immune system at the present time. (Ref. 1, pp. 451, 469, 471)

8 Collagen Vascular Disorders

DIRECTIONS: Each of the questions or incomplete phrases below is followed by five suggested answers or completions. Select the **one** that is best in each case.

189. The acute systemic form of juvenile rheumatoid arthritis is characterized by all of the following EXCEPT
    A. it accounts for 50% of the children with JRA
    B. it is associated with high fever and chills
    C. actue symptoms may precede joint symptoms by as much as six months
    D. a salmon colored morbilliform rash
    E. hepatosplenomegaly is seen in approximately one-third of cases

190. The monoarticular form of JRA is characterized by all of the following EXCEPT
    A. it accounts for approximately 30% of cases of JRA
    B. iridocyclitis is a significant systemic manifestation and occurs in as many as 25% of patients
    C. small joints are commonly involved
    D. fatigue and low-grade fever are not prominent symptoms
    E. painless swelling of the joints is common

191. Polyarticular JRA is characterized by all of the following EXCEPT
  - **A.** involvement of multiple joints, including fingers and toes
  - **B.** systemic manifestations, including iridocyclitis, which are rare
  - **C.** severe pain, erythema, and warmth which are very common
  - **D.** usually symmetrical joint involvement, with the large joints involved first
  - **E.** limitation of joint motion, which occurs early

192. Which of the following statements regarding laboratory studies in JRA is true?
  - **A.** ESR is frequently normal in all forms of JRA
  - **B.** In a child with monoarticular arthritis, there is an increased likelihood of development of eye disease with a positive antinuclear antibody titer
  - **C.** The majority of children with acute systemic JRA have normal WBC count during active disease
  - **D.** Rheumatoid factor is commonly positive
  - **E.** Positive rheumatoid factor and antinuclear antibody titer in the same patient are pathognomonic of JRA

193. Which of the following does NOT characterize systemic lupus erythematosus?
  - **A.** Tests for autoantibodies are frequently positive
  - **B.** Family members of patients with SLE have increased incidence of hypergammaglobulinemia, rheumatoid factor, and ANA
  - **C.** Skin manifestations of SLE without systemic disease are common in children
  - **D.** Severe arthritis is present only infrequently, and deforming arthritis is rare
  - **E.** Renal involvement is common at some time during the course of the disease

194. Which of the following statements regarding laboratory tests does NOT characterize SLE?
    A. Antinuclear antibody (ANA) is the single most important test
    B. ANA is a specific test for SLE
    C. LE preparation is less frequently positive in chldren than adults
    D. A positive LE prep is more specific for the diagnosis of SLE than is a positive ANA test
    E. Creatinine clearance is a useful indicator of the severity of renal involvement

195. All of the following are major criteria in the diagnosis of dermatomyositis in childhood EXCEPT
    A. progressive symmetric weakness of peripheral muscle groups
    B. evidence of necrosis of type I and type II muscle fibers
    C. elevation of skeletal muscle enzymes in serum
    D. characteristic heliptrope rash with periorbital edema
    E. scaly erythematous rash over the dorsum of the hands

DIRECTIONS: Each set of lettered headings below is followed by a list of numbered words or phrases. For each numbered word or phrase select

A   if the item is associated with **A** only,
B   if the item is associated with **B** only,
C   if the item is associated with both **A** and **B**,
D   if the item is associated with neither **A** nor **B**.

Table 3 Modified Jones Criteria

Major Manifestations	Minor Manifestations	Supporting Evidence of Strep Infection
Carditis	Fever	Recent scarlet fever
Polyarthritis	Arthralgia	Positive throat culture
Chorea	Previous rheumatic fever	Increased ASO
Erythema marginatum	Positive acute phase reactants such as ESR, C-reactive protein, leukocytosis	
Subcutaneous nodules	Prolonged P-R interval	

The presence of two major or of one major and two minor manifestations supported by evidence of recent streptococcal infection indicates a high probability of acute rheumatic fever.

Questions 196–200 Study Table 3.

    A.   Kawasaki syndrome
    B.   Acute rheumatic fever
    C.   Both
    D.   Neither

196.   Congestive heart failure may be a feature

197.   Penicillin is effective therapy in reducing complications

198.   Arthritis is a common feature

199.   Coronary artery aneurysms are a serious component of the disease

200.   Prednisone may be indicated

DIRECTIONS: For each of the questions or incomplete statements below, **one or more** of the answers or completions given is correct. Select

A   if only **1**, **2**, and **3** are correct,
B   if only **1** and **3** are correct,
C   if only **2** and **4** are correct,
D   if only **4** is correct,
E   if all are correct.

201. In systemic lupus erythematosus
    1. anti-DNA antibodies are common
    2. steroids have no place in treatment
    3. immune complexes deposit in the nephron
    4. serum complement determinations are of little value

202. Henoch–Schönlein syndrome (anaphylactoid purpura) may be characterized by
    1. arthritis, with or without effusion
    2. gastrointestinal bleeding
    3. variable skin rash
    4. renal involvement which may progress to chronic renal disease

203. Clinical manifestations of systemic lupus erythematosus include
    1. hepatitis
    2. nephritis
    3. iritis
    4. psychosis

Collagen Vascular Disorders
Answers and Comments

189. A. The acute systemic form of JRA accounts for approximately 20% of the cases. (Ref. 1, p. 432)

190. C. Knees, ankles, and elbows are the joints commonly involved. Small joints of the hands are conspicuously spared. (Ref. 1, p. 432)

191. C. Severely painful, red, hot joints are unusual in polyarticular JRA. (Ref. 1, p. 432)

192. B. ESR and WBCs are frequently normal in patients with monoarticular, polyarticular, and pauciarticular arthritis but are elevated in the majority of children with acute systemic JRA. Rheumatoid factor is rarely positive in children with JRA. (Ref. 1, p. 433)

193. C. Discoid lupus is rare in children. (Ref. 1, p. 436)

194. B. A positive test for ANA may be present in chronic active hepatitis, Sjögren syndrome, and rarely JRA. (Ref. 1, p. 436)

195. A. Muscle weakness is found in the limb girdle groups and anterior neck flexors. (Ref. 1, p. 438)

196. C. Congestive heart failure may be seen in both of these
197. D. diseases. Penicillin is indicated in rheumatic fever if
198. C. there is still evidence of strep infection. It has no effect
199. A. on the sequelae once acute rheumatic fever is occurring,
200. B. and it has no therapeutic value in Kawasaki syndrome.
Prednisone may be indicated in acute rheumatic fever, in addition to aspirin, but it is contraindicated in Kawasaki disease because it may increase the frequency of aneurysm formation. Arthritis may be a feature of both. (Ref. 3, pp. 155, 499)

201. B. Systemic lupus erythematosus is an autoimmune disease in which anti-DNA antibodies are formed, and renal immune complex deposition occurs. Only rarely may patients with SLE be managed without steroids. The level of serum C3 is a valuable guide to the activity of the disease. (Ref. 1, p. 437)

202. E. Anaphylactoid purpura is a syndrome that may include: arthritis with or without effusion, GI bleeding, a variable skin rash, and nephritis that can progress to chronic renal disease in some patients. (Ref. 2, p. 577)

203. E. The clinical manifestations of SLE are the result of the widespread vasculitis that accompanies this disorder. The liver, eye, brain, and kidney may all be involved. (Ref. 2, p. 575)

9 Bacterial and Viral Infections

DIRECTIONS: Each of the questions or incomplete statements below is followed by five suggested answers or completions. Select the **one** that is best in each case.

---

204. Endotoxin is characterized by all of the following EXCEPT
  A. it is a lipopolysaccharide component of the outer membrane of the organism
  B. it may promote a consumption coagulopathy by activating the clotting sequence
  C. it fixes complement directly via the alternate pathway
  D. it produces hypothermia
  E. it is one of the main surface antigens of gram-negative organisms

205. The organism most commonly associated with neonatal bacterial disease is
  A. *Staphylococcus aureus*
  B. group B beta-hemolytic streptococci
  C. *Listeria monocytogenes*
  D. *Escherichia coli*
  E. *Pseudomonas*

206. The most common bacterial organism associated with meningitis in infants and children is
   A. *Diplococcus pneumoniae*
   B. *Neisseria meningitidis*
   C. group A beta-hemolytic streptococcus
   D. *Haemophilus influenzae*
   E. group B beta-hemolytic streptococcus

207. Which of the following statements does NOT characterize bacterial meningitis in young infants?
   A. Only specific feature may be bulging of the anterior fontanelle
   B. Nuchal rigidity is commonly present
   C. *H. influenzae* is the most common organism
   D. Papilledema is rarely seen
   E. Poor feeding is common

208. Viral meningitis is characterized by all of the following EXCEPT
   A. CSF cell count may show transient predominance in polymorphonuclear WBCs early in the course
   B. CSF sugar is elevated
   C. CSF protein may be moderately elevated
   D. CSF findings are similar to lead encephalitis
   E. predominant cytology is mononuclear

209. Subdural effusions complicating meningitis are associated with all of the following EXCEPT
   A. extremely rare in meningococcal meningitis
   B. persistent vomiting recurring after initial clinical improvement
   C. most commonly accompany infection caused by *H. influenzae* and *D. pneumoniae*
   D. patients frequently show signs of cerebral damage
   E. recovery of 2 ml or more of xanthochromic fluid with a protein content exceeding by 40 mg that of the spinal fluid·

210. Concerning infection due to *Corynebacterium diphtheriae*, which of the following statements is FALSE?
    A. Myocarditis is a common lesion and the changes are degenerative rather than inflammatory
    B. Bacteria usually remain on surface lesions of respiratory systems and rarely cause bacteremia
    C. Complications due to the toxins may occur as late as six weeks after the initial infection
    D. Primary nasal involvement is usually seen in older children and adults
    E. Incubation period is usually between two to five days

211. The most common manifestation of disseminated gonorrhea in adolescents and adults is
    A. myocarditis
    B. meningitis
    C. hemorrhagic skin lesions
    D. pyelonephritis
    E. arthritis

212. Which of the following statements is FALSE regarding gonococcal infections?
    A. Prior infections usually confer protective immunity
    B. Associated with production of local and systemic antibody as well as cell-mediated response
    C. Predilection for infecting mucosal surfaces lined by columnar as opposed to stratified epithelium
    D. pH of vaginal mucus and thickness of mucosa are important modifiers in susceptibility to infection
    E. Symptoms usually appear within one week of infection

213. Infection with *H. influenzae* is characterized by all of the following EXCEPT
  A. it is the most common bacterial meningitis in young children
  B. synergy with certain respiratory viruses may be important in colonization production of local respiratory disease
  C. 95% of invasive strains are type B
  D. the nonencapsulated organism is associated with disease more often than the encapsulated form
  E. facial cellulitis is more common than pyarthrosis

214. Acute epiglottitis due to *H. influenzae* type B is characterized by all of the following EXCEPT
  A. sore throat
  B. dysphagia
  C. stridor
  D. position of ease is supine with chin extended
  E. fever

215. A differential diagnosis of meningococcal disease would include all of the following EXCEPT
  A. Coxsackie type A9 viral infection
  B. rickettsial disease
  C. ECHO viral infection
  D. atypical measles
  E. adenoviral infection

Recent outbreaks of pertussis in England have stressed the importance of proper, complete immunizations for all children. Table 4 lists the current recommendations of the American Academy of Pediatrics.

Table 4 Recommended Schedule for Active Immunization of Normal Infants and Children

Recommended Age	Vaccine(s)	Comments
2 mo	DTP,[1] OPV[2]	Can be initiated earlier in areas of high endemicity
4 mo	DTP, OPV	2-mo interval desired for OPV to avoid interference
6 mo	DTP (OPV)	OPV optional for areas where polio might be imported (e.g., some areas of Southwest United States)
12 mo	Tuberculin Test[3]	May be given simultaneously with MMR at 15 mo
15 mo	Measles, Mumps, Rubella (MMR)[4]	MMR preferred
18 mo	DTP, OPV	Consider as part of primary series—DTP essential
4–6 yr[5]	DTP, OPV	
14–16 yr	Td[6]	Repeat every 10 years for lifetime

[1]DTP—Diphtheria and tetanus toxoids with pertussis vaccine.

[2]OPV—Oral, attenuated poliovirus vaccine contains poliovirus types 1, 2, and 3.

[3]Tuberculin test—Mantoux (intradermal PPD) preferred. Frequency of tests depends on local epidemiology. The Committee recommends annual or biennial testing unless local circumstances dictate less frequent or no testing (see Tuberculosis for complete discussion).

[4]MMR—Live measles, mumps, and rubella viruses in a combined vaccine (see text for discussion of single vaccines versus combination).

[5]Up to the seventh birthday.

[6]Td—Adult tetanus toxoid (full dose) and diphtheria toxoid (reduced dose) in combination.

For all products used, consult manufacturer's brochure for instructions for storage, handling, and administration. Biologics prepared by different manufacturers may vary, and those of the same manufacturer may change from time to time. The package insert should be followed for a specific product.

Reprinted with permission from *Pediatrics, 59* (5), Part 2, May 1977. Copyright American Academy of Pediatrics 1982.

216. Which of the following is considered to be effective pro-
phylaxis against meningococcal infections among close
contacts?
A. Penicillin
B. Rifampin
C. Sulfonamide
D. Tetracycline
E. Erythromycin

217. Which of the following is NOT considered characteristic of
pertussis (Table 4)?
A. May be seen early in life owing to a lack of maternal
antibodies
B. The catarrhal stage precedes the paroxysmal stage
C. The paroxysmal cough may last for one to four weeks
D. The peripheral WBC is usually significantly elevated
with a shift to polymorphonuclear leukocytes
E. Incubation period is between five and ten days

218. Regarding pathogenesis of tuberculosis, which of the following is FALSE?
A. Tuberculin hypersensitivity develops in the host four
to eight weeks after infection, and the skin test becomes
positive
B. The greatest risk for progression of primary complex
with occurrence of meningitis and miliary disease is
during the first 12 months after the primary infection
C. Skeletal lesions appear within two to four years of the
primary lesion
D. Renal lesions appear early within two to three years of
the primary infection
E. The nodal component of the primary complex shows
less tendency to heal completely than the parenchymal
focus

219. Primary tuberculosis is characterized by all of the following EXCEPT
  A. an incubation period of two to eight weeks
  B. the majority of cases are innocuous with healing and calcification of Ghon complex occurring as early as six months
  C. the most common symptoms of progressive disease are cough, fever, and night sweats
  D. involvement of bronchial wall by enlarging lymph nodes is a rare complication of primary complex
  E. the skin test is nonreactive for eight weeks after the initial infection

220. The treatment of choice for lymph node disease due to nontubercular mycobacterial organism is
  A. complete excision
  B. isoniazid (INH)
  C. INH, paraaminosalicyclic acid (PAS)
  D. rifampin
  E. ethambutol

221. Which of the following does NOT characterize salmonellosis (nontyphoid fever)?
  A. The most common form is the gastroenteric type
  B. Rose spots, splenomegaly and leukopenia occur in the *Salmonella paratyphi* form
  C. *Salmonella typhimurium* is the most common organism found in salmonella gastroenteritis
  D. Among the localized infections due to metastatic infection, meningitis is the most common
  E. Patients with sickle disease are particularly susceptible to osteomyelitis

222. Which of the following is NOT characteristic of enteropathogenic *E. coli* enteritis?
  A. Leukocytosis
  B. Watery stools
  C. Stools that contain neither blood nor pus
  D. Principal complications are secondary infections chiefly of the respiratory tract, the meninges, or the skin
  E. Intestinal mucosa usually shows no ulceration

223. Staphylococcal food poisoning is usually manifested by all of the following EXCEPT
    A. colicky abdominal pain
    B. little if any fever
    C. severe, watery mucoid diarrhea
    D. onset of symptoms a few hours after eating infected food
    E. it is rarely fatal

224. Scarlet fever is associated with all of the following findings EXCEPT
    A. infection due to erythrogenic toxin producing group A beta-hemolytic streptococci
    B. punctate erythematous lesions on the palate
    C. early onset (24 to 48 hours) of erythematous punctiform rash
    D. heavy involvement of rash over face
    E. Pastia's lines

225. Group B beta-hemolytic streptococcal disease in the immediate newborn period differs from the delayed onset disease in all of the following EXCEPT
    A. meningitis is the most common manifestation
    B. maternal factors are more common, i.e., premature labor, maternal perinatal fever
    C. mortality is higher in the immediate period
    D. onset is more sudden
    E. clinical course is more rapid

226. Pathologic features that distinguish the syphilis of infancy and early childhood from that of later life include all of the following EXCEPT
    A. interstitial fibrosis of liver and spleen
    B. pneumonia consisting of increased connective tissue infiltrating the lung
    C. increased incidence of cardiovascular disease
    D. tissue alteration leading to allergic type lesion such as interstitial keratitis
    E. scarring of lips and nose tissues

227. Which of the following is FALSE in regard to immunology and serodiagnosis of childhood syphilis?
    A. Maternal IgG may be transplacentally transmitted to the fetus
    B. Nonspecific antibody to syphilis may also be found in infectious mononucleosis, vaccinic, varicella, and SLE
    C. Antibodies are of the IgM and IgG types
    D. Transplacentally transferred antibody will produce a positive serologic test for syphilis (STS) but not a positive *Treponema pallidum* immobilization test (TPI)
    E. Transplacentally transferred antibody may be equal to but not greater than the mother's

228. Varicella is characterized by all of the following EXCEPT
    A. one attack usually confers lifelong immunity
    B. maternal varicella antibody is transplacentally passed when a pregnant woman gets varicella
    C. incubation period ranges from 11 to 20 days
    D. if it occurs during the first ten days of life it may result in disseminated infection
    E. varicella is generally much more severe in children than in adults

229. Which of the following is NOT characteristic of varicella?
    A. Lesions appear in crops over a period of three to five days
    B. Distribution of lesions is predominantly on the extremities as compared to the trunk
    C. The peripheral blood picture is essentially unchanged
    D. Primary varicella pneumonia is uncommon
    E. Prodromal period is mild, and symptoms may be absent

230. Congenital cytomegalovirus (CMV) is characterized by all of the following EXCEPT
    A. approximately 95% of affected infants are asymptomatic
    B. often the only physical finding is a general failure to thrive or increased irritability
    C. major complications of the infection are sequelae involving the CNS
    D. paraventricular cerebral calcification is more common than hepatosplenomegaly
    E. petechial rash on first day after birth suggestive of disease

231. Which of the following statements regarding acquired cytomegaloviral mononucleosis is FALSE?
    A. Atypical lymphocytosis is common
    B. May be associated with a maculopapular rash following ampicillin administration
    C. Usually heterophil antibody positive
    D. The cytomegalovirus IgM (FA) test is positive in CMV and infectious mononucleosis presumably because EBV and CMV share common antigens
    E. Hepatomegaly and mildly abnormal liver function tests are found

232. Exanthema subitum (roseola infantum) is best distinguished from rubella by which of the following?
    A. Height and duration of fever preceding the rash
    B. Character of the rash
    C. Location of lymphadenopathy
    D. Peripheral WBC
    E. Response to treatment

233. The most common viral agent associated with gastroenteritis in infants and young children is
    A. ECHO virus
    B. Rotavirus
    C. Coxsackie virus
    D. Norwalk virus
    E. coronavirus

234. Which of the following does NOT accurately characterize the clinical picture of viral hepatitis in children?
   A. Onset is often abrupt
   B. Anorexia and nausea and vomiting are common preicteric symptoms
   C. Generalized jaundice most often precedes the color change in urine owing to excess bilirubin
   D. Massive necrosis of hepatic parenchymal cells is rare
   E. Constipation and diarrhea occur occasionally and with equal frequency

Table 5 Serologic Markers of Viral Hepatitis

Condition	IgM Anti HA	HB$_s$Ag	HB$_e$Ag	Anti HBe	Anti HB$_c$	Anti HB$_s$
Acute HA	+	−	−	−	−	−
Early acute HB	−	+	+	−	−	−
Acute HB	−	+	+	−	+	−
Chronic HB	−	+	+/−	+/−	+	+/−
Past infection with HBV	−	−	−	−	+	+

An understanding of the serologic markers in hepatitis is important. Study the table above.

235. Which of the following statements differentiating type A hepatitis from type B hepatitis (Table 5) is FALSE?
   A. Onset is more abrupt with type A
   B. Fever is more frequent with type A
   C. Inapparent infections more common with type B
   D. Higher proportion of urticarial rashes and joint manifestations with type A
   E. Type B has been associated with, and is presumably a cause of, polyarteritis and glomerulonephritis

236. Which of the following statements is FALSE regarding hepatitis B surface antigen (HBsAg) testing?

    A. Becomes positive one to two months prior to onset of symptoms

    B. A positive test for HBsAg that becomes negative in convalescence is diagnostic of type B hepatitis

    C. Positive at onset of jaundice in majority of cases

    D. Positivity is not an index of carrier state

    E. Used as basis for screening blood donors for the carrier state

237. Hepatitis B virus can be transmitted from man to man by all of the following EXCEPT

    A. in urine

    B. in saliva

    C. transplacentally

    D. venereally

    E. in feces

238. Which of the following statements concerning the virology and epidemiology of herpes simplex virus (HSV) is FALSE?

    A. HSV type 2 primarily infects genital sites

    B. Recrudescenses of infections occur in individuals with circulating HSV antibodies

    C. Infectious virus can be demonstrated in sensory ganglia

    D. Incubation period for neonates with herpetic infection is an average of one week

    E. Genital HSV-2 infection in pregnant women has been found to be the major source of virus for the newborn

239. Regarding the clinical manifestations of HSV infections, which of the following is FALSE?

    A. The lips are the most common site for HSV-1 recurrences, but are infrequently the site for primary infection

    B. The oral cavity is the most common site of infection in children

    C. Eczema herpeticum is most often caused by a primary HSV infection

    D. The most common site of genital infection in females with HSV-2 is the labia

    E. Asymptomatic HSV infections in the newborn are infrequent

240. HSV infection of the CNS is characterized by all of the following EXCEPT
    A. most isolates from the brain of individuals beyond the newborn age are HSV-1
    B. HSV meningitis is primarily caused by HSV-1
    C. HSV meningitis is difficult to differentiate from other causes of aseptic meningitis
    D. brain biopsy is the only certain way to diagnose HSV encephalitis
    E. HSV-2 is more readily recoverable from the CSF than is HSV-1

241. The epidemiology of Epstein-Barr virus (EBV) infection is characterized by all of the following EXCEPT
    A. it is most often acquired during childhood
    B. infection usually occurs without clinically recognizable symptoms
    C. mononucleosis usually occurs during infection in adolescence and early adulthood
    D. there is a higher rate of infection among the upper socioeconomic groups
    E. the role of reactivated virus in the genesis of the disease or in transmission has not yet been clarified

242. Infectious mononucleosis is clinically manifested by all of the following EXCEPT
    A. the classic picture is rarely seen in toddlers and young children infected with EBV
    B. heterophil agglutination is sometimes not detected in young children
    C. splenomegaly is observed in approximately 50% of patients during the second and third week of illness
    D. hepatomegaly and liver tenderness are found in a low percentage of patients, as are elevated liver enzymes
    E. generalized lymphadenopathy of gradual onset is characteristic

243. Laboratory findings in infectious mononucleosis are characterized by all of the following EXCEPT

A. the height of the heterophil antibody titer is not related to clinical severity of the disease

B. heterophil antibodies cross-react with other EBV associated antigens

C. the heterophil antibody titer in mononucleosis serum is not significantly reduced by guinea pig kidney absorption, but is completely absorbed by beef erythrocytes

D. during acute mononucleosis there is marked increase of the total serum IgM

E. during the first week of illness the WBC count may be normal or there may be leukopenia due to granulocytopenia

244. Which of the following does NOT distinguish the infectious mononucleosis caused by EBV from that caused by cytomegalovirus?

A. Atypical lymphocytosis with fever

B. Negative heterophil antibodies

C. Cervical adenopathy

D. Tonsillar exudate

E. Sore throat

245. Acute lymphocytosis can be differentiated from infectious mononucleosis due to EBV by all of the following EXCEPT

A. adenopathy

B. splenomegaly

C. atypical lymphocytes

D. lymphocytosis

E. heterophil antibodies

246. The epidemiology and pathology of respiratory syncytial viral infection is characterized by all of the following EXCEPT

    A. it is the most important viral respiratory pathogen of infancy and childhood

    B. its peak incidence occurs in the first year of life with most serious illness occurring in the first six months

    C. maternal serum antibody is protective

    D. evidence that reinfection with RSV frequently triggers wheezing attacks in children with chronic asthma

    E. replication of virus in initial infection occurs in oro- and nasopharynx

247. Clinical features of RSV may be described by all of the following EXCEPT

    A. RSV bronchiolitis usually manifested by wheezing and reaches its peak severity in 48 to 72 hours

    B. CO_2 retention may be presumed to begin when the respiratory rate surpasses 60 per minute

    C. distinction between RSV bronchiolitis and RSV pneumonia is usually easily made

    D. RSV disease in younger infants is generally worse than in older children

    E. RSV pneumonia generally resolves spontaneously in the course of a few weeks

248. Which of the following does NOT characterize influenza infections?

    A. Incubation period is short, usually one to three days

    B. Physical and x-ray evidence of pneumonia is generally the rule rather than the exception in influenza illness

    C. Localized pneumonia is often caused by secondary infection with pneumococci and *Staphylococcus aureus*

    D. Routine laboratory studies are usually within normal limits with the exception of elevation of ESR

    E. Physical findings in the typical case are few

249. The pathogenesis and epidemiology of measles are characterized by all of the following EXCEPT
    A. although less than 1% of patients develop signs and symptoms of encephalomyelitis, about 50% show EEG changes
    B. measles virus has not been recovered from the CSF or CNS tissue of patients with encephalomyelitis
    C. single attack confers lifelong immunity
    D. the disease is most communicable during the rash stage
    E. nearly all patients have demonstrable circulating serum antibodies by the second day of rash

250. Which of the following is FALSE regarding measles immunization?
    A. The attenuated vaccines provide an infection that is communicable
    B. Secondary bacterial infections and neurologic complications that accompany natural or modified measles do not occur following a vaccination
    C. Serious complications may occur in children exposed to natural measles after having been vaccinated years before with killed vaccine
    D. Given at the appropriate time, live vaccine provides 95% prophylactic efficacy
    E. It may diminish cutaneous delayed hypersensitivity reaction to tuberculoprotein

251. The epidemiology of mumps is characterized by all of the following EXCEPT
    A. mumps is endemic at all times
    B. orchitis and meningoencephalitis may occur in the absence of parotitis
    C. transplacental immunity probably accounts for the infrequency of mumps in the first six months after birth
    D. the incubation period may last as long as a month
    E. it is more communicable than measles and varicella

252. The clinical manifestations of mumps are characterized by
     all of the following EXCEPT
     A. unilateral parotid involvement is more frequent
     B. orchitis is very rare in childhood
     C. submaxillary or sublingual glands may be the only sal-
         ivary glands involved
     D. meningoencephalitis may be the only evidence of
         mumps
     E. pancreatitis occurs much less frequently in children
         than in adults

253. Which of the following does NOT characterize the epide-
     miology of Coxsackie viral infection?
     A. Group B viruses are associated with epidemic myalgia
     B. Group A viruses are associated with myocarditis and
         pericarditis
     C. Group A viruses are usually associated with herpangina
     D. Sporadic acute illness with exanthems is associated with
         groups A and B
     E. Both groups are associated with hepatitis

254. Herpangina is manifested by all of the following EXCEPT
     A. it is caused by Coxsackie group A
     B. clinical laboratory findings are normal
     C. lesions are most commonly located on gingiva and buc-
         cal mucosa
     D. headache and abdominal symptoms are common
     E. recovery is usually uncomplicated

255. The hand-foot-mouth disease of Coxsackie viral infection is
     characterized by all of the following EXCEPT
     A. it is caused by group B virus
     B. constitutional symptoms are usually mild
     C. routine laboratory results are usually within normal
         limits
     D. skin manifestations include vesicles in mouth, hands,
         and feet accompanied by a maculopapular rash on
         extremities
     E. complications are very rare

256. Of the following statements concerning rubella, which is FALSE?
    A. The exanthem is variable and may be scarlatiniform in appearance
    B. It is not as highly contagious as measles
    C. Arthritis is uncommon in children
    D. Thrombocytopenia as a complication is very rare
    E. Adenopathy may persist for weeks.

257. The most common manifestation of congenital rubella in the neonatal period is
    A. congenital heart disease
    B. thrombocytopenic purpura
    C. cataracts
    D. neurologic defects
    E. hepatosplenomegaly

258. Which of the following statements concerning congenital rubella is FALSE?
    A. The risk of fetal abnormalities associated with maternal rubella infection late in the second trimester or later is minimal
    B. The infant may remain chronically infected for months after birth
    C. IgM is the dominant rubella antibody at one year of age
    D. The presence of rubella specific IgM reflects in utero antibody production by the fetus
    E. Isolation of virus from the blood is rare

259. Which of the following statements concerning trachoma and inclusion conjunctivitis agent is FALSE?
    A. Trachoma infection is limited to the eyes
    B. Inclusion conjunctivitis agent resides in the genital tract of adults
    C. Conjunctival scarring and corneal vascularization and opacification may occur in trachoma
    D. Infection with inclusion conjunctivitis agent responds poorly to antibodies and may result in corneal scarring
    E. Classified as members of the psittacosis group

260. Of the human rickettsioses, which is NOT associated with a generalized rash?
   A. Epidemic typhus
   B. Rocky mountain spotted fever
   C. Rickettsial pox
   D. Q fever
   E. Murine typhus

261. Which of the following statements concerning human rickettsioses is NOT true?
   A. Commonly used antibiotics suppress, but do not destroy, the organisms
   B. Viable pathogenic organisms may be found in lymph nodes of patients convalescing from typhus and Rocky mountain spotted fever
   C. Weil-Felix reaction is the most reliable test for rickettsial disease
   D. Organisms are highly infective and require intracellular milieu for growth
   E. Pathologic lesion of the exanthematous rickettsioses includes generalized involvement of small blood vessels

262. Rocky mountain spotted fever is clinically manifested by all of the following EXCEPT
   A. the exanthem is evidence of vasculitis involving small vessels
   B. CNS involvement is greater in patients with Rocky mountain spotted fever than in those with other rickettsial diseases
   C. thrombocytopenia is an uncommon finding
   D. the rash usually begins on extremities
   E. CSF is generally normal except for mild lymphocytic pleocytosis

263. Q fever most often mimics which of the following diseases?
   A. Atypical pneumonia
   B. Varicella
   C. Primary herpetic infection
   D. Rocky mountain spotted fever
   E. Viral gastroenteritis

Proper treatment of a potential rabies patient is important. Study this table.

Table 6 Rabies Postexposure Prophylaxis Guide, March 1980

The following recommendations are only a guide. In applying them, take into account the animal species involved, the circumstances of the bite or other exposure, the vaccination status of the animal, and presence of rabies in the region. Local or state public health officials should be consulted if questions arise about the need for rabies prophylaxis.

Animal species	Condition of animal at time of attack	Treatment of exposed person[1]
Domestic		
dog and cat	healthy and available for ten days of observation	none, unless animal develops rabies[2]
	rabid or suspected rabid	RIG[3] and HDCV[4]
	unknown (escaped)	consult public health officials. If treatment is indicated, give RIG[3] and HDCV[4]
Wild		
skunk, bat, fox, coyote, raccoon, bobcat, and other carnivores	regard as rabid unless proven negative by laboratory tests[5]	RIG[3] and HDCV[4]
Other		
livestock, rodents, and lagomorphs (rabbits and hares)	Consider individually. Local and state public health officials should be consulted on questions about the need for rabies prophylaxis. Bites of squirrels, hamsters, guinea pigs, gerbils, chipmunks, rats, mice, other rodents, rabbits, and hares almost never call for antirabies prophylaxis.	

[1] All bites and wounds should immediately be thoroughly cleansed with soap and water. If antirabies treatment is indicated, both rabies immune globulin (RIG) and human diploid cell rabies vaccine (HDCV) should be given as soon as possible, regardless of the interval from exposure.

[2] During the usual holding period of 10 days, begin treatment with RIG and vaccine (preferably with HDCV) at first sign of rabies in a dog or cat that has bitten someone. The symptomatic animal should be killed immediately and tested.

[3] If RIG is not available, use antirabies serum, equine (ARS). Do not use more than the recommended dosage.

[4] If HDCV is not available, use duck embryo vaccine (DEV). Local reactions to vaccines are common and do not contraindicate continuing treatment. Discontinue vaccine if fluorescent-antibody (FA) tests of the animal are negative.

[5] The animal should be killed and tested as soon as possible. Holding for observation is not recommended.

Reprinted from *CDC, Morbidity and Mortality Weekly Report (MMWR)*, June 13, 1980: Vol. 29, No. 23.

DIRECTIONS: Each group of questions below consists of five lettered headings, followed by a list of numbered words, phrases, or statements. For each numbered word, phrase, or statement, select the **one** lettered heading that is most closely associated with it. Each lettered heading may be selected once, more than once, or not at all.

    A. Rabies (Study Table 6)
    B. Tularemia
    C. Leptospirosis
    D. Brucellosis
    E. *Mycoplasma pneumoniae*

264. Associated with ingestion of infected milk products

265. Erythromycin may be an effective therapy

266. Variable incubation period from 10 days to more than a year

267. Zoonosis transmitted by contact with infected rabbits

268. Fluid and electrolyte changes, especially hyponatremia, may be important complications

    A. Hepatitis A
    B. Hepatitis B
    C. Hepatitis non-A, non-B
    D. All of the above
    E. None of the above

269. Transfusion related

270. Immune serum globulin effective in prevention

271. Abrupt onset in children, with shorter course

272. Transmission via breastmilk

273. Chronic active hepatitis a common complication

Bacterial and Viral Infections
Answers and Comments

204. D. Endotoxic action causes neutrophils to liberate a small protein (leukocyte pyrogen) that acts on anterior hypothalamic nuclei, causing fever. (Ref. 1, p. 481)

205. B. Group B streptococci along with the slightly less common *E. coli* are currently considered the major organisms. (Ref. 1, p. 511)

206. D. Following *H. influenzae, D. pneumoniae* and *N. meningitidis* are the most common. (Ref. 1, p. 515)

207. B. Nuchal rigidity is most often absent. (Ref. 1, p. 516)

208. B. With the exception of mumps meningoencephalitis, CSF sugar is almost always normal. (Ref. 1, p. 1705)

209. D. The majority of patients in whom an abnormal volume of fluid is obtained have no clinical sign of cerebral damage. (Ref. 1, p. 1718)

210. D. Nasal diphtheria is seen particularly in infants and very young children and is usually very mild. (Ref. 1, p. 527)

211. E. During the phase of bacteremia a migratory polyarthritis is typical. (Ref. 1, p. 532)

212. A. Prior infection does not confer immunity. The significance of the immunological activity is not well understood. (Ref. 1, p. 530)

213. D. The pathogenicity of invasive diseases is related not only to the age of the host but also to the presence of type B capsule. (Ref. 1, p. 533)

214. D. A child almost always assumes a sitting position, leaning forward with chin extended. (Ref. 1, p. 535)

215. E. Adenoviral disease is usually not associated with petechial and maculopapular eruptions. (Ref. 1, p. 539)

216. B. Although little experience exists in the use of rifampin in children, it is useful in eradicating carriage of meningococci. (Ref. 1, p. 541)

217. D. Total WBC count is usually in the range of 25000 to 40000 with a predominance of small mature lymphocytes. These appear in the circulation as a result of the discharge of the marginal pool under influence of lymphocyte promoting factor of *B. pertussis*. (Ref. 1, p. 541)

218. D. Renal lesions occur late and rarely before five years after infection. (Ref. 1, p. 569–574)

219. D. Nodal involvement with the bronchial wall is common, occurring with a frequency of up to 20%. (Ref. 1, p. 569–574)

220. A. Most strains are resistant to drug therapy. Excision is the treatment of choice when nodes are easily accessible. (Ref. 1, p. 582)

221. D. Arthritis is the most common localized infection. Osteomyelitis, cystitis, meningitis, endocarditis, and soft tissue abscesses have been reported. (Ref. 1, p. 547)

222. A. Leukocytosis is not characteristic of enteropathogenic *E. coli* enteritis. (Ref. 1, p. 552)

223. C. Diarrhea does not always accompany staphylococcal food poisoning, but when it does it is relatively mild. (Ref. 1, p. 555)

224. D. The face is usually spared from the rash, with the heaviest concentration in the flexural creases. (Ref. 1, p. 558)

225. A. Pneumonia and sepsis are more common in immediate period; meningitis is more common in delayed onset disease. (Ref. 1, p. 512)

226. C. Cardiovascular involvement in childhood disease is rare, contrasted with a 15% incidence, most commonly aortitis, in adults. (Ref. 1, p. 562)

227. D. Both antibodies tested in STS and TPI behave similarly. Both disappear from the infant and are unmeasureable in most infants in eight weeks and in all by 12 weeks of age. (Ref. 1, p. 561)

228. E. Varicella, like many other viral infections, is much more severe in adults than in children. (Ref. 1, p. 611)

229. B. The distribution of the lesions is predominantly centripetal. (Ref. 1, p. 612)

230. D. Clinical manifestations most frequently seen among symptomatic newborns in order of decreasing frequency are hepatosplenomegaly, jaundice, purpura, microcephaly, chorioretinitis, and paraventricular cerebral calcification. (Ref. 1, p. 590)

231. C. Patients with CMV mononucleosis are always heterophil antibody negative. (Ref. 1, p. 591)

232. A. Roseola is characterized by sudden onset of high fever lasting for several days, and with defervescence the rubellalike rash appears. (Ref. 1, p. 614)

233. B. Rotavirus is a reolike virus that rarely causes diarrhea in adults. (Ref. 1, p. 615)

234. C. The brown discoloration of urine is often the first clue to the diagnosis of viral hepatitis. (Ref. 1, p. 618)

235. D. Not only are joint manifestations more common with type B infections, but polyarteritis and glomerulonephritis are more common also. (Ref. 1, p. 618)

236. D. HBsAg positively is an index of carrier state that supervenes in 5 to 10% of overt cases. (Ref. 1, p. 619)

237. E. The antigenic and structural integrity are rapidly lost in the presence of intestinal and bacterial enzymes. (Ref. 1, p. 619)

238. C. Infectious virus cannot be demonstrated with sensory ganglia; however by using special cultivation methods of the ganglia, it can be reactivated. (Ref. 1, p. 585–588)

239. D. The most common site of involvement is the cervix. (Ref. 1, p. 587)

240. B. HSV meningitis is primarily caused by HSV-2, is rarely found in children, but may be encountered in adolescents and in immunologically compromised individuals. (Ref. 1, p. 588)

241. D. In lower socioeconomic groups approximately 80% of children have antibody by the age of six years. (Ref. 1, p. 592)

242. D. Although hepatomegaly is found in only 10% of patients elevated levels of SGOT and serum LDH are seen in the majority of patients, and these persist for weeks to months after the disease. (Ref. 1, p. 592)

243. B. Heterophil antibodies do not cross react with any known EBV associated antigens and the manner in which EBV infection induces these antibodies is not known. (Ref. 1, p. 593)

244. A. The characteristics of CMV mononucleosis are atypical lymphocytosis, fever, and hepatosplenomegaly. (Ref. 1, p. 593)

245. D. Absolute lymphocytosis is characteristic, but the lymphocytes are small and mature. (Ref. 1, p. 594)

246. C. Serum maternal antibody provides no protection. It has been postulated that in the absence of secretory antibody, local or systemic cellular immunity, serum antibody may lead to exacerbation of RSV infection. (Ref. 1, p. 595)

247. C. Rales and wheezing may be found in both entities so that the distinction is often arbitrary. (Ref. 1, p. 595)

248. B. Clinical and x-ray evidence of pneumonia is unusual in the uncomplicated case of influenza. (Ref. 1, p. 598)

249. D. The disease is most communicable during the viremia stage (first 7 to 10 days after exposure). In addition to being recoverable from the respiratory tract it can also be found in nasopharyngeal secretions, urine, and blood. (Ref. 1, p. 621)

250. A. Attenuated vaccines are not associated with communicability. (Ref. 1, p. 625)

251. E. Mumps is less communicable than measles, varicella, or pertussis. (Ref. 1, p. 625)

252. A. Bilateral involvement occurs with approximately 70% of cases. (Ref. 1, p. 626)

253. A. Group B viruses have most often been associated with cardiac disease. (Ref. 1, p. 604)

254. C. Lesions commonly located on the fauces, soft palate, and uvula. (Ref. 1, p. 605)

255. A. The hand-foot-mouth disease is caused by Coxsackie virus A5 or A16. (Ref. 1, p. 605)

256. D. Many patients have a slight but definite decrease in platelets during the course of uncomplicated rubella, and it usually occurs within one week after onset of rash. (Ref. 1, p. 632)

257. B. All of the others occur but may not be manifested until after the neonatal period. (Ref. 1, p. 634)

258. C. Except in rare cases, IgG is usually the dominant rubella antibody found in infants at one year of age. (Ref. 1, p. 635)

259. D. Inclusion conjunctivitis responds to topical therapy, and although the untreated infection can persist for months, it leaves without residue. (Ref. 1, p. 524)

260. D. In Q fever, cutaneous involvement is not apparent, and the disease generally is confined to the lungs and liver. (Ref. 1, p. 641)

261. C. Specific serologic reactions using rickettsial antigens in complement fixation agglutination, or neutralization tests, are more reliable. (Ref. 1, p. 640)

262. C. Thrombocytopenia is commonly found and is a result of peripheral sequestration or of an injury to the platelets. (Ref. 1, p. 643)

263. A. Respiratory manifestations usually predominate and there is no rash. (Ref. 1, p. 645)

264. D. Brucellosis is associated with the ingestion of infected
265. E. milk products, and is prevented by pasturization. Eryth-
266. A. romycin may be effective therapy for *Mycoplasma* in-
267. B. fections. Rabies has a very variable incubation period,
268. C. probably related to site of the bite, amount of inoculum, and a variety of host factors. Tularemia, or "rabbit fever" is most commonly seen in hunters. Leptospirosis can result in severe electrolyte changes, in addition to jaundice, hemorrhagic manifestations, and renal involvement. (Ref. 3, pp. 546, 547, 559, 573, 580)

269. B, C. Hepatitis A is transmitted by the fecal oral route, tends
270. D. to have a more abrupt onset, and is preventable in
271. A. close contacts by administration of immune serum
272. E. globulin. Hepatitis B is present in many body secre-
273. E. tions, and is most commonly transmitted by transfusion, sharing of needles among drug users, and rectal intercourse among homosexual men. It is preventable by use of hepatitis B immune globulin or vaccination. Hepatitis non-A, non-B is believed to be largely transfusion associated, but it may be indicated to give immune serum globulin to contacts. Chronic active hepatitis is an uncommon complication in children. Although hepatitis B surface antigen has been demonstrated in breastmilk, transmission via this route is unlikely and has never been documented. (Ref. 2, p. 784)

10 Mycotic and Parasitic Diseases

DIRECTIONS: Each of the questions or incomplete statements below is followed by five suggested answers or completions. Select the **one** that is best in each case.

---

274. Infection with *Blastomyces dermatitidis* is characterized by all of the following EXCEPT
    A. the lungs are the primary site of infection
    B. the majority of patients will have positive complement fixation tests
    C. chronic cutaneous blastomycosis is the most common form of North American blastomycosis and is the presenting complaint of most patients
    D. it is responsive to amphotericin B
    E. the pulmonary form is difficult to distinguish from active tuberculosis

275. The clinical picture of coccidioidomycosis may be associated with all of the following EXCEPT
    A. the primary nonfatal form is usually associated with respiratory disease that may be asymptomatic
    B. a negative coccidioidin skin test in a patient with erythema nodosum usually eliminates the possibility of coccidioidomycosis
    C. negative serologic tests virtually rule out the chronic disseminated form of the disease
    D. organisms may be found in sputum, gastric washings, CSF, and pleural or peritoneal fluid
    E. amphotericin B is indicated in primary coccidioidomycosis

276. The primary acute form of histoplasmosis is characterized by all of the following EXCEPT
    A. the primary site is the lungs
    B. it is usually mild and often asymptomatic
    C. a histoplasmin skin test is positive three to five weeks after infection
    D. amphotericin B therapy is indicated
    E. subpleural tubercles are formed

277. Cryptococcosis is associated with all of the following EXCEPT
    A. it is seen most frequently in patients with serious underlying disease
    B. infection is usually acquired by inhalation
    C. CNS involvement is a rare complication
    D. pulmonary infection may be a common manifestation and may be asymptomatic
    E. its primary source is avian excrement

278. Which of the following signs or symptoms does NOT usually characterize ascariasis?
    A. Urticaria
    B. Cough with hemoptysis
    C. Eosinophilia
    D. Vague abdominal pain
    E. Hepatomegaly

279. Visceral larva migrans is associated with all of the following EXCEPT

A. humans are not usually the hosts of the dog ascarid, *Toxocara canis*

B. the larvae migrate most often to the lungs

C. lesions are necrotizing or granulomatous and heavily infiltrated with eosinophils

D. the most characteristic clinical picture is of hepato-megaly, eosinophilia, fever, cough, and wheezing

E. hyperglobulinemia

280. Enterobiasis (*Enterobius vermicularis*) is associated with all of the following EXCEPT

A. it does not require a host other than the human and does not require soil for maturation

B. eosinophilia is a common manifestation

C. ova are infrequently seen in the stool

D. there is no portal migration

E. there is no pulmonary migration

281. Hookworm disease (*Necator americanus*) is characterized by all of the following EXCEPT

A. migration through the lungs is indispensable to development

B. a period of time in the soil is necessary for development of larvae

C. pulmonic infiltrative disease with consolidation is common

D. a common abnormality is microcytic hypochromic anemia

E. growth failure may be seen in some patients

282. Amebiasis (*Entamoeba histolytica*) is associated with all of the following EXCEPT
   A. transmission is by ingestion of cysts
   B. trophozoites emerge from cysts as a result of the action of digestive enzymes
   C. intestinal bacteria are essential to production of intestinal lesions by trophozoites
   D. intestinal lesions remain superficial
   E. liver abscess is a frequent complication

283. The etiology and epidemiology of toxoplasmosis are characterized by all of the following EXCEPT
   A. toxoplasma is a coccidian parasite of cats
   B. infection may be acquired by ingestion of infective oocysts in the soil or tissue cysts in raw meat
   C. the fetus is at greatest risk from transplacental transmission during the first and second trimester
   D. worldwide distribution is seen
   E. responsible for habitual abortions

284. Which of the following is LEAST often encountered in acute congenital toxoplasmosis seen during the immediate postnatal period?
   A. Intracerebral calcifications
   B. Thrombocytopenic purpura
   C. Severe jaundice
   D. Hepatosplenomegaly
   E. Chorioretinitis

DIRECTIONS: Each set of lettered headings below is followed by a list of numbered words or phrases. For each numbered word or phrase select

A if the item is associated with **A** only,
B if the item is associated with **B** only,
C if the item is associated with both **A** and **B**,
D if the item is associated with neither **A** nor **B**.

A. Blastomycosis
B. Actinomycosis
C. Both
D. Neither

285. Has a pulmonary form of infection

286. Most commonly seen as a chronic cutaneous infection

287. Penicillin is the drug of choice

288. Amphotericin B is the drug of choice

289. Can be seen on microscopic smears of specimens

A. *E. histolytica*
B. *Giardia lamblia*
C. Both
D. Neither

290. Creates deep ulcers in colon wall

291. A protozoan

292. Pulmonary migration is a part of the life cycle

293. Frequent asymptomatic colonization

294. Can form visceral abscesses

Mycotic and Parasitic Diseases
Answers and Comments

274. B. Apparently less than 50% of the sera from patients with proved blastomycosis give a positive complement fixation test. Furthermore, since cross-reaction between North American blastomycosis and histoplasmosis is not uncommon, a single serologic examination must be interpreted with caution. (Ref. 1, p. 650)

275. E. The primary form of the disease usually requires no therapy, since it is self-limited. Intravenous amphotericin B is indicated in the disseminated form. (Ref. 1, p. 654)

276. D. In the usual mild self-limited attacks no specific antifungal therapy is indicated. (Ref. 1, p. 657)

277. C. CNS infection is a common manifestation, and meningitis is regarded as the most frequent cause of mycotic meningitis. (Ref. 1, p. 656)

278. E. Migration through the portal system and liver usually does not cause significant pathology. (Ref. 1, p. 660)

279. B. Migration is usually to the liver, less frequently to the lungs, kidneys, heart, brain, eye, and striated muscle. (Ref. 1, p. 661)

280. B. Eosinophilia is seldom observed in enterobiasis. (Ref. 1, p. 662)

281. C. Pulmonary consolidation during lung phase is distinctly uncommon. (Ref. 1, p. 663)

282. D. In severe infections, the colonic ulcers may extend to the peritoneal surface with perforation. (Ref. 1, p. 684)

283. E. Transmission to the fetus occurs only if the primary infection occurs during pregnancy. Responsibility for habitual abortion is no longer regarded as valid. (Ref. 1, p. 702)

284. **A.** Intracerebral calcification is usually found in the sub-acute form, and is not observed until sometime after birth. (Ref. 1, p. 704)

285. **C.** Actinomycosis and blastomycosis can appear as primar-
286. **A.** ily pulmonary infections. The diagnosis can be suggested
287. **B.** by examination of smears of material from the lesions.
288. **A.** Penicillin is the drug of choice for actinomycosis, while
289. **C.** amphotericin B is used in blastomycosis. Blastomycosis most commonly appears as a chronic cutaneous infection, while actinomycosis does not. (Ref. 1, p. 647, 650)

290. **A.** *Entamoeba* can be a very invasive organism, causing
291. **C.** deep colonic ulcers and abscesses in many organs in-
292. **D.** cluding the brain and the liver. It can be found in symp-
293. **C.** tomless carriers and it does not have a pulmonary
294. **A.** migration. *Giardia* is also a protozoan but it is of low virulence and does not form abscesses. It can also be found in asymptomatic carriers, but it lives mainly in the small bowel and not the colon. Like *Entamoeba*, it does not exhibit pulmonary migration. (Ref. 2, pp. 835, 837)

11 Endocrine and Metabolic Disorders

DIRECTIONS: Each of the questions or incomplete statements below is followed by five suggested answers or completions. Select the **one** that is best in each case.

---

295. Phenylketonuria is a metabolic disorder in which
   A. melanocytes cannot form melanin
   B. phenylalanine cannot be converted to tyrosine
   C. histidine cannot be converted to urocanic acid
   D. valine cannot be deaminated
   E. methylmalonyl-CoA cannot be metabolized

296. All of the following are characteristic of maple syrup urine disease EXCEPT
   A. infants appear well at birth
   B. early manifestations include feeding difficulty, irregular respirations, or loss of Moro reflex
   C. convulsions are a rare complication
   D. symptoms begin three to five days after birth
   E. the disease is caused by branched-chain ketoaciduria

117

297. Homocystinuria is characterized by all of the following EXCEPT
    A. it is the most common inherited disorder of amino acid metabolism
    B. the disorder involves the sulfur-containing amino acids
    C. most patients are mentally retarded
    D. death usually occurs before age one year
    E. spontaneous arterial and venous thromboembolic phenomena are prominent

298. All of the following are true of Lesch-Nyhan syndrome EXCEPT
    A. severe mental retardation
    B. cerebral palsy
    C. choreoathetosis
    D. self-destructive biting
    E. renal aminoglycinuria

299. All of the following are correct statements regarding galactosemia EXCEPT
    A. it is inherited as an autosomal recessive disorder
    B. the infant usually appears normal at birth, and the clinical signs appear after initiation of milk feedings
    C. hepatomegaly is a late sign
    D. lethargy and hypotonia are frequent findings
    E. the signs may resemble sepsis

300. Hereditary fructose intolerance is characterized by all of the following EXCEPT
    A. symptomatology when fructose is ingested in the diet
    B. hypoglycemia, tremors, disorientation are present
    C. chronic ingestion resembles galactosemia
    D. enzyme defect is a deficiency of hepatic aldolase
    E. treatment involves using cortisone because of its gluconeogenic effect

301. The most common heritable lipid disease is
    A. Gaucher disease
    B. metachromatic leukodystrophy
    C. Niemann–Pick disease
    D. Tay–Sachs disease
    E. Fabry disease

302. In the diagnostic evaluation of a child with short stature, psychosocial dwarfism is being considered. Which of the following is NOT associated with this disorder?
    A. Psychologically disturbed child with emotional deprivation
    B. Short stature, polyphagia, polydipsia, and polyuria
    C. Shyness and temper tantrums
    D. Delayed skeletal development
    E. Diagnosis proved by dramatic response to growth hormone

303. The blood ADH level is high in all of the following EXCEPT
    A. nephrotic syndrome
    B. pain, and after anesthesia
    C. after cardiac surgery
    D. with the use of most pain medications
    E. cirrhosis

304. All of the following are characteristic of congenital adrenal hyperplasia EXCEPT
    A. deficient production of cortisol starts about two weeks after birth
    B. excessive secretion of adrenal androgens in the female fetus causes masculinization of the external genitalia
    C. acute adrenal crisis of salt-losing form is due to absence of secretion of aldosterone
    D. infants have poor appetites and fail to gain weight
    E. excessive loss of sodium results in severe water loss and dehydration

305. Which of the following is NOT characteristic of adrenogenital syndrome?
    A. Hypersecretion of adrenal androgens causes symptoms of virilism and increased protein anabolism
    B. Virilizing adrenal tumors are rarely palpable but can displace kidney from its normal position
    C. Urinary 17 ketosteroids are decreased
    D. Virilizing adrenal tumors do not produce excessive amounts of cortisol
    E. In boys and girls, muscles are well developed

306. All of the following are characteristic of congenital hypothyroidism EXCEPT
    A. infants are born with little or no evidence of thyroid hormone deficiency
    B. classic facies is a result of accumulation of myxedema in subcutaneous tissues and tongue
    C. prolonged hypothyroidism results in muscular hypotonia and mental defects
    D. T4 values are low and thyroid stimulating hormone concentrations are high in newborns
    E. the best guide to measure effectiveness of therapy is to observe physical changes

307. The presence of a goiter at birth is usually the result of
    A. ingestion of goitrogenic substances by the mother
    B. congenital hypothyroidism
    C. severe peroxidase deficiencies
    D. thyroglossal duct abnormalities
    E. thyroiditis congenita

308. All of the following are characteristic of juvenile thyrotoxicosis EXCEPT

    A. it occurs almost exclusively as a consequence of hyperfunctioning nodules

    B. onset is insidious with increasing nervousness, palpitations, and increased appetite

    C. rarely do children show a weight increase with the onset of disease

    D. behavior abnormalities and declining school performance are prominent

    E. signs and symptoms are similar to those produced by a hyperactive sympathetic nervous system

309. Pathognomonic signs of hypoglycemia in a five-year-old are

    A. sweating, pallor, and fatigue

    B. pallor, tremors, and nervousness

    C. bradycardia, nervousness, and fever

    D. drowsiness, eye-rolling, and sweating

    E. none of the above

310. Relatively common causes of diabetes insipidus include all of the following EXCEPT

    A. tumors of suprasellar and chiasmatic regions, particularly craniopharyngiomas

    B. reticuloendothelioses

    C. encephalitis, sarcoidoisis, leukemia

    D. genetic faults

    E. operative procedures in the pituitary or hypothalamic regions

---

DIRECTIONS: Each group of questions below consists of five lettered headings followed by a list of numbered words, phrases, or statements. For each numbered word, phrase, or statement, select the **one** lettered heading that is most closely associated with it. Each lettered heading may be used once, more than once, or not at all.

A. Phenylketonuria
B. Isovaleric acidemia
C. Alkaptonuria
D. Hartnup disease
E. Propionic acidemia

311. Mental and physical retardation, osteoporosis, and periodic thrombocytopenia

312. Associated with the odor of "sweaty feet"

313. Arthritis and ochronosis

314. Caused by the absence of the hepatic enzyme phenylalanine hydroxylase

315. Defect in the transport of tryptophan by the intestinal mucosa and renal tubule

316. High frequency among fair-skinned, blue-eyed blondes with this disorder

A. Gaucher disease
B. Hunter syndrome
C. Tay–Sachs disease
D. Acute intermittent porphyria
E. Hurler syndrome

317. Seen exclusively in males

318. Very high incidence in persons with Ashkenazi Jewish ancestry

319. Associated with cataracts

320. An abnormality in heme metabolism

321. Caused by β glucosidase deficiency

322. Caused by N-acetylgalactosaminidase

    A. Thromboembolic episodes
    B. Cataracts
    C. Recurrent abdominal pain
    D. Diaper turns black
    E. Hypoglycemia

323. Galactosemia

324. Nesidioblastosis

325. Alcaptonuria

326. Lactase deficiency

327. Homocystinemia

Endocrine and Metabolic Disorders
Answers and Comments

295. B. As a result of the inability to convert phenylalanine to tyrosine there is an accumulation of phenylpyruvic acid, which is excreted in the urine. In classic PKU the major clinical problem is mental retardation. The fundamental biochemical defect in PKU is the absence of phenylalanine hydroxylase. (Ref. 1, p. 260)

296. -C. Convulsions are characteristic of the disease. The infant develops opisthotonos and generalized muscular rigidity. Signs of decerebrate rigidity are seen prior to death, which occurs within two to four weeks. (Ref. 1, p. 264)

297. A. Homocystinuria is the second most common inherited disorder of amino acid metabolism. In this regard, PKU occurs with greater frequency. (Ref. 1, p. 269)

298. E. The metabolic defect in Lesch-Nyhan syndrome is hyperuricemia. Children with this disorder may excrete over 600 mg/day of uric acid. The disease is transmitted as an X-linked recessive, involving the activity of the enzyme hypoxanthine guanine phosphoribosyl transferase. (Ref. 1, p. 277)

299. C. In galactosemia there is early evidence of liver involvement. Hepatomegaly is a common and constant finding. Jaundice is frequent and death may occur early from hepatic failure. (Ref. 1, p. 280)

300. E. Treatment of hereditary fructose intolerance includes control of (1) IV administration of glucose-containing fluids for the acute symptoms and (2) avoidance of fructose- and sucrose-containing foods for the long term. (Ref. 1, p. 282)

301. D. Tay–Sachs disease occurs in persons of Ashkenazi Jewish ancestry; gene frequency is one in 60 persons. The incidence is much less frequent in offspring of non-Jewish ancestry. The disorder is the result of the absence of N-acetylgalactosaminidase. (Ref. 1, p. 316)

302. E. The diagnosis of psychosocial dwarfism can only be proved by removing the child from his noxious environment, and observing more rapid growth in a favorable environment. Rapid growth spurts are reported when these children are relocated in a more advantageous environment. (Ref. 1, p. 1472)

303. D. Blood ADH is high in shock, nephrotic syndrome, cirrhosis, pain, after surgical procedures, and diseases characterized by hypoproteinemia and edema. ADH levels are increased following the administration of vincristine. (Ref. 1, p. 1478)

304. A. Congenital adrenal hyperplasia is a congenital disease. The deficiency of production of cortisol starts during fetal life. (Ref. 1, p. 1490)

305. C. Urinary neutral 17-ketosteroids are usually greatly elevated. The elevation is due in part to the increase in dehydroepiandrosterone (DHA), which represents 50% or more of the total urinary 17-KS. Virilizing adrenal tumors show no suppression of plasma androgen urinary 17-KS during two dexamethasone suppression tests. (Ref. 1, p. 1490)

306. E. The best guide to measure success of therapy is to monitor the circulating levels of T4 and TSH. History and physical examination are important, but they may not reveal mild hypo- or hyperthyroidism. (Ref. 1, p. 1526)

307. A. In the United States the most common cause of neonatal goiter is the maternal ingestion of large doses of iodides during pregnancy. The iodides are usually found in expectorants (prescribed for asthma), or for treatment of maternal thyrotoxicosis. Other goitrogens include: thioureas, sulfonamides, and hematinic medications containing cobalt. (Ref. 1, p. 1524)

308. A. Juvenile thyrotoxicosis (Graves disease) occurs almost exclusively as a result of diffuse thyroid hyperplasia rather than hyperfunctioning nodules. Girls are affected six times more frequently than boys, and there is a sharp increase in the disease during early adolescence. (Ref. 1, p. 1532)

309. E. There are no pathognomonic signs of hypoglycemia in children. The signs are very mercurial and differ from child to child. The child may exhibit variations of sweating, pallor, fatigue, tachycardia, and nervousness caused by an excessive secretion of epinephrine. CNS signs include headache, irritability, behavioral changes, confusion, seizures, and coma. (Ref. 2, p. 1421)

310. D. Diabetes insipidus results from the lack of antidiuretic hormone arginine vasopressin. Any lesion that damages the neurohypophysial unit may result in diabetes insipidus. Tumors and infiltrative disorders can do this, as well as basal skull fractures. Only in a minority of instances is the condition due to heredity. Autosomal dominant and X-linked recessive inheritance is known. (Ref. 2, p. 1437)

311. E. Phenylketonuria is caused by the absence of the hepatic
312. B. enzyme phenylalanine hydroxylase and the frequency is
313. C. high among fair skinned and blue-eyed persons. Patients
314. A. with isovaleric acidemia are said to have the odor of
315. D. "sweaty feet" because of the accumulation of short-
316. A. chained fatty acids. Hartnup disease is caused by a defect in the transport of tryptophan in the intestinal mucosa and renal tubule. Infants with propionic acidemia frequently present with mental and physical retardation, osteoporosis, and periodic thrombocytopenia. Alkaptonuria is characterized by the accumulation and excretion in the urine of homogentisic acid and its oxidation products. The slow accumulation of the black polymer of homogentisic acid in cartilage produces a black discoloration: alkaptonuric ochronosis. (Ref. 2, pp. 424–432)

317. B. Tay–Sachs disease is caused by N-acetylgalatosamini-
318. C. dase deficiency and is of very high incidence among per-
319. E. sons of Ashkenazi Jewish ancestry. Hunter syndrome is
320. D. an X-linked recessive disorder and is thus seen only in
321. A. males and is not associated with cataracts, while patients
322. C. with Hurler syndrome have cataracts. Gaucher disease is caused by a beta-glucosidase deficiency. Acute intermittent porphyria is caused by a defect in heme metabolism. (Ref. 1, pp. 313, 316, 337, 339, 342)

323. **B, E.** Galactosemia is associated with cataracts and hypo-
324. **E.** glycemia. If left untreated, it can produce liver damage
325. **D.** and severe mental retardation. Nesidioblastosis is a
326. **C.** recessive disorder which results in proliferation of pan-
327. **A.** creatic beta cells, resulting in recurrent hypoglycemia.
Homogentisic acid accumulates in alcaptonuria, a disorder of tyrosine metabolism. Its oxidation causes the diaper to turn black,
and arthritis and a black discoloration of cheeks, scelerae, ears
and nose are complications in later life. Lactase deficiency results
in diarrhea, distension, and abdominal pain. Thromoembolic phe-
nomena, ectopia lentis, and mental retardation are found in homocystinemia, a disorder of methionine metabolism. (Ref. 2,
pp. 427, 446, 1423)

12 Circulatory System

DIRECTIONS: Each of the questions or incomplete statements below is followed by five suggested answers or completions. Select the **one** that is best in each case.

---

328. All of the following statements concerning the auscultation of heart sounds in children are true EXCEPT

- **A.** a third heart sound is common in normal children
- **B.** the second heart sound is due to closure of the semilunar valves
- **C.** the first heart sound is reduced in intensity when cardiac output is increased
- **D.** a fourth heart sound is generally associated with significant obstruction to ventricular ejection
- **E.** the origin of the normal first heart sound is debatable

329. Which of the following characteristics most clearly differentiates the venous hum from patent ductus arteriosus?

- **A.** Position auscultation on the chest wall
- **B.** Heard in both systole and diastole
- **C.** Venous hum murmur is always of low intensity
- **D.** Exaggeration or disappearance of murmur by position of head
- **E.** Changes in intensity with exercise

330. In which of the following situations is further clinical evaluation indicated?
    A. A newborn with a heart rate of 130
    B. A two-year-old with a heart rate of 110
    C. A newborn with a pulse rate of 90 during sleep
    D. A two-month-old infant with a pulse rate of 130
    E. A crying two-month-old with a pulse rate of 260

331. Which of the following statements concerning the determination of arterial blood pressure is true?
    A. With cuff technique blood pressure is normally lower in the leg than arm
    B. Flush blood pressure is equal to diastolic pressure
    C. Blood pressure varies little with the age of the child until the late teens
    D. Exercise or excitement may raise systolic pressure of children as much as 40 to 50 mmHg above usual levels
    E. Use of a cuff that is too large will result in false high blood pressure readings

332. The cardiac defect associated with maternal and fetal rubella infection is
    A. aortic valvular insufficiency
    B. pulmonic valve insufficiency
    C. patent ductus arteriosus
    D. mitral valve insufficiency
    E. dextrocardia and pulmonic stenosis

333. In the management of paroxysmal dyspneic attacks in patients with tetralogy of Fallot, all of the following pertain EXCEPT
    A. attacks are preventable by avoidance of excitement and exercise
    B. knee chest position may give relief
    C. O_2 administration may alleviate symptoms
    D. propranolol has been used successfully in some patients
    E. attacks are most prominent during the first two years of life

334. In the neonate with isolated transposition of the great arteries all of the following are true EXCEPT
    A. recognition of cyanosis may be delayed in the first few days of life
    B. normal birthweight
    C. murmurs are absent in the majority in the first few days of life
    D. tachypnea is present
    E. massive cardiomegaly is common

335. Patients with Ebstein's disease have all of the following characteristics EXCEPT
    A. downward displacement of an abnormal tricuspid valve into the right ventricle
    B. may have no symptoms until adulthood
    C. both systolic and diastolic murmurs
    D. small right atrium and enormous right ventricle
    E. large, saillike anterior tricuspid leaflet

336. Hypoplastic left heart syndrome may be accompanied by all of the following symptoms EXCEPT
    A. dyspnea
    B. hepatomegaly
    C. cyanosis
    D. femoral pulses increased and brachial pulses decreased
    E. metabolic acidosis

337. The signs and symptoms of an infant with a moderate ventricular septal defect include all of the following EXCEPT
    A. tachypnea and dyspnea
    B. feeding difficulties
    C. slow growth
    D. higher risk for pulmonary infection
    E. intermittent cyanosis

338. The most common clinical manifestation of ventricular septal defect is
    A. signs of congestive heart failure in the first week of life
    B. small septal defects with trivial left-to-right shunt
    C. cyanosis
    D. chronic bronchitis
    E. moderate left-to-right shunting at the atrial level

Table 7 Prevention of Bacterial Endocarditis in Patients with Rheumatic Fever or Congenital Heart Disease

Procedure	Recommended Regimen
Dental procedures with bleeding tonsillectomy, adenoidectomy, bronchoscopy	Penicillin G (30,000 U/kg up to a maximum adult dose of 1,000,000 U) mixed with procaine penicillin G (600,000 U) and given IM 30–60 min before procedure, followed by penicillin V (< 28 kg, 250 mg; > 28 kg, 500 mg) orally q 6 hr × 8
OR	Penicillin V (< 28 kg, 1 gm 30–60 min before procedure, then 250 mg q 6 hr × 8; double the dose for > 28 kg)
Genitourinary or gastrointestinal surgery or instrumentation	Aqueous penicillin G (30,000 U/kg to maximum adult dose of 2,000,000 U) or ampicillin (50 mg/kg up to maximum adult dose of 1 g) IM or IV
PLUS	Gentamicin (children 2 mg/kg, adults 1.5 mg/kg maximum for both 80 mg IM or IV) or streptomycin (20 mg/kg, up to maximum adult dose of 1 gm IM)

339. All of the following are important in the prevention of sub-acute bacterial endocarditis (Table 7) in patients with ventricular septal defect EXCEPT
   A. the condition of the teeth
   B. the use of antibiotics for dental extraction
   C. the use of antibiotics for tonsillectomy
   D. early use of antibiotics for bacterial infections of the respiratory tract
   E. monthly injections of long-acting penicillin

DIRECTIONS: Each group of questions below consists of five lettered headings, followed by a list of numbered words, phrases, or statements. For each numbered word, phrase, or statement, select the **one** lettered heading that is most closely associated with it. Each lettered heading may be selected once, more than once, or not at all.

Table 8 Principal Diagnostic Criteria for Mucocutaneous Lymph Node Syndrome

Fever, persisting for more than five days

Conjunctival injection

Changes in the mouth consisting of:
  Erythema, fissuring and crusting of the lips
  Strawberry tongue
  Diffuse oropharyngeal erythema

Erythematous rash

Enlarged lymph nodes

Changes in the extremities consisting of:
  Induration of hands and feet
  Erythema of palms and soles
  Desquamation of finger and toetips about two weeks after onset

Transverse grooves across fingernails two to three months after onset

Questions 340–344 Match the following signs or symptoms with the appropriate clinical problem (Table 8).

    A. Changing murmur, fever, splenomegaly
    B. Pericardial effusion
    C. Cerebral thrombosis
    D. Heart failure in early infancy
    E. Coronary artery thrombosis

340. Kawasaki disease

341. Tetralogy of Fallot

342. Viral myocarditis

343. *H. influenzae* meningitis

344. Small VSD

DIRECTIONS: For each of the questions or incomplete statements below, **one or more** of the answers or completions given is correct. Select

    A   if only **1, 2,** and **3** are correct,
    B   if only **1** and **3** are correct,
    C   if only **2** and **4** are correct,
    D   if only **4** is correct,
    E   if all are correct.

---

345. Changes in cardiac output and distribution of blood flow shortly after birth include
    1. rapid rise in cardiac output per kilogram of body weight over the first three months
    2. sharp fall in pulmonary blood flow
    3. rapid rise in right ventricular output
    4. rapid fall in pulmonary arterial pressure

346. Factors that are thought to contribute to maintaining the patency of the ductus arteriosus are
    1. increased pulmonary vascular resistance secondary to hypoxia
    2. high arterial oxygen tension
    3. prostaglandin
    4. acetylcholine

347. The echocardiograph can be used to
    1. diagnose myocardial infarction
    2. determine the presence of a pericardial effusion
    3. distinguish a pathologic from an innocent murmur
    4. demonstrate the relationships of the great vessels to other cardiac structures

348. In second degree AV block
    1. every atrial impulse is conducted to the ventricle
    2. the outcome is usually fatal
    3. tachycardia frequently occurs
    4. there is almost always underlying heart disease

349. Cardiac lesions that can cause left-to-right shunts include
1. patent ductus arteriosus
2. anomalous origin of left coronary artery
3. ventricular septal defect
4. sinus of Valsalva fistula

350. In ventricular septal defect
1. the murmur is generally harsh and of plateau type
2. the smaller the defect, the greater the likelihood of spontaneous closure
3. a mid-diastolic rumble may occur
4. right-to-left shunting of blood is not part of the natural course of the disease

351. Metabolic derangements that may affect myocardial function include
1. Pompe disease
2. Hunter syndrome
3. hemachromatosis
4. cystinosis

Circulatory System
Answers and Comments

328. C. The first heart sound is increased in high cardiac output states. This sound is related to events occurring in early systole, and factors other than closure of the AV valves contribute. These include the rapid rise in isometric contraction. (Ref. 2, p. 1100)

329. D. The venous hum will change with positioning changes of the head or light compression over the veins in the neck. (Ref. 2, p. 1104)

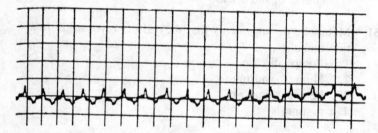

Figure 7 Tracing of paroxysmal atrial tachycardia.

330. E. A pulse rate of 260 in the presence of vigorous crying is considered cause for further investigation and observation. The infant may be experiencing an arrhythmia, such as paroxysmal atrial tachycardia (Fig. 7). (Ref. 2, p. 1100)

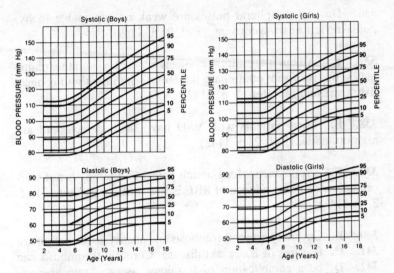

Figure 8 Percentiles of blood pressure management, right arm, seated. (Reprinted with permission from Blumenthal, S. et al.: Report of the task force on blood pressure in children. *Pediatrics* 59:797 (suppl.), 1977.)

331. D. Blood pressure is normally higher in the legs; flush pressure is an index of mean arterial pressure. Blood pressure varies considerably with age (Fig. 8), and nomograms are available. A cuff that is too large for the extremity will produce falsely low readings. (Ref. 2, pp. 1252–1253)

332. C. Patent ductus arteriosus and pulmonary arterial branch stenosis are associated with congenital rubella. (Ref. 2, p. 412)

333. A. Attacks may be spontaneous and unpredictable. (Ref. 2, p. 1123)

334. E. Significant cardiomegaly is unusual in the neonate with isolated transposition of the great arteries. (Ref. 2, p. 1131)

335. D. The right atrium is enormous, and the size of the right ventricle is reduced in patients with Ebstein disease. (Ref. 2, p. 1136)

336. D. All peripheral pulses are weak or impalpable in hypoplastic left heart syndrome. (Ref. 2, p. 1139)

337. E. All but intermittent cyanosis may occur, and the infants may suffer recurrent pulmonary infections with or without congestive heart failure. (Ref. 2, p. 1142)

338. B. Most patients with VSD have small defects and are asymptomatic. (Ref. 2, p. 1142)

339. E. Prophylactic, long-acting penicillin therapy is not warranted, since the incidence of SBE is low in these patients. (Ref. 2, p. 1143)

340. E. Coronary artery thrombosis and aneurysm formation are
341. C. features of Kawasaki disease. Cerebral thrombosis can
342. D. be a complication of tetralogy, as can brain abscess.
343. B. Viral myocarditis, especially due to Coxsackie B viruses
344. A. can cause heart failure in early infancy. *H. influenzae* meningitis has recently been found to be associated with apparently benign pericardial effusions. While the incidence is not as high as with valvular lesions, SBE can be a complication of VSDs. (Ref. 3, pp. 135, 499, 535)

345. D. Shortly after birth there is an initial rise in cardiac output, but over the next three months it falls slowly. The RV output remains approximately the same. Pulmonary arterial blood flow rises sharply and pulmonary arterial pressure falls. (Ref. 1, p. 1232)

346. B. The ductus arteriosus is kept open by prostaglandins and by hypoxia-induced pulmonary hypertension. The ductus is closed by high arterial oxygen tensions and acetylcholine. (Ref. 1, p. 1233)

347. C. The echocardiograph can be used to detect the presence of pericardial fluid and to demonstrate the relationships of the great vessels to each other and other structures. The echocardiogram cannot diagnose MI nor can it distinguish murmurs. (Ref. 1, p. 1250)

348. D. In second degree AV block there is almost always underlying heart disease, and therefore it deserves thorough investigation. The ventricular rate is usually slow, and the block is at the level of the AV node and His system, thus sometimes blocking beats generated in the atria from reaching the ventricle. The condition is not usually fatal since the advent of treatment with pacemakers. (Ref. 1, p. 1265)

349. E. All of the cardiac lesions listed have the creation of left-to-right shunting of blood as a pathological feature. (Ref. 1, p. 1281)

350. A. In VSD the murmur is of a harsh quality and of the plateau type, but if the ratio of pulmonary to systemic flow is 2:1 then a diastolic rumble can occur. Many of the smaller VSDs close spontaneously. If the shunt is significant and unrelieved by surgery, then pulmonary hypertension can occur, with a resulting right-to-left shunting of blood. (Ref. 1, p. 1289)

351. E. The myocardium is damaged by glycogen in Pompe disease, by hemosiderin deposition in hemochromatosis, by cystine crystals in cystinosis, and by degeneration in the mucopolysaccharidosis (Hunter and Hurler syndromes). (Ref. 1, p. 1347)

13 Nervous System

DIRECTIONS: Each of the questions or incomplete statements below is followed by five suggested answers or completions. Select the **one** that is best in each case.

---

352. Chorea is more often associated with
    A. idiosyncracy to phenothiazines
    B. forms of encephalitis
    C. hepatolenticular degeneration
    D. dystonia musculorum
    E. rheumatic fever

353. Probably the most frequent cause of hydrocephalus is
    A. spina bifida with meningomyelocele
    B. postinflammatory or posttraumatic obstruction
    C. Dandy-Walker syndrome
    D. neoplasm (glioma in the third ventricle)
    E. Arnold Chiari malformation

354. All of the following are true statements regarding anencephaly EXCEPT
   A. it is the most common CNS malformation incompatible with life
   B. it is six times more common in whites than in blacks
   C. it is three times more common in males than females
   D. the mother often has hydramnios
   E. the diagnosis can be made prepartum by x-ray of the abdomen

355. Which of the following is NOT true of increased intracranial pressure associated with a brain tumor?
   A. Headache site is of value in localizing tumor
   B. Cranial enlargement can result from obstructive hydrocephalus
   C. Vomiting tends to occur on arising
   D. Double vision can result from sixth nerve palsy
   E. Papilledema may not be present

356. All of the following are associated with cerebellar astrocytoma EXCEPT
   A. no age is exempt, but peak incidence is from 5 to 8 years of age
   B. the majority of patients are symptomatic less than two months prior to diagnosis
   C. there are signs and symptoms of increased intracranial pressure
   D. ataxia predominates on one side
   E. nystagmus and head tilt are present

357. Medulloblastoma is usually NOT associated with
   A. signs and symptoms similar to cerebellar astrocytoma
   B. onset usually more acute than with cerebellar astrocytoma
   C. seizures
   D. rapid course
   E. poor prognosis

358. Which of the following is NOT characteristic of craniopharyngioma?
   A. Evidences of increased intracranial pressure
   B. Presence of visual defects
   C. Endocrine dysfunctions, diminished pituitary activity
   D. Growth retardation
   E. Diabetes insipidus in over 50% of cases

359. The most frequent symptoms of intraspinal tumors in children are
   A. disturbance of gait and posture
   B. pain
   C. decreased deep tendon reflexes
   D. enuresis and encopresis
   E. a bruit over the vertebral column

360. Pseudotumor cerebri is characterized by all of the following EXCEPT
   A. increased intracranial pressure
   B. convulsions and impaired mentation
   C. blurred vision and diplopia
   D. florid papilledema and abducens nerve paresis
   E. no consistent signs of neurologic dysfunction

361. A seven-year-old child presents with seizures, depressed sensorium, focal motor deficits, and signs of circulatory stasis. Temperature is elevated. An abscess of the nose is found. The most likely diagnosis is
   A. fat embolism
   B. periarteritis nodosa
   C. venous thromboses
   D. dissecting cerebral aneurysm
   E. pseudotumor cerebri

362. Regarding extradural hematoma, all of the following are true EXCEPT
    A. it is most common in children less than two years of age
    B. it is the most lethal complication of head injury. The untreated mortality is 100%
    C. there is no mechanism for absorption of an extradural hemorrhage and, therefore, there is a rapid rise in intracranial pressure
    D. treatment is surgical
    E. untreated cases survive only two to three days

363. A 14- and six-per-second positive spike dysrhythmia during light sleep on EEG suggests
    A. grand mal seizure
    B. absence seizure (petit mal)
    C. hypsarhythmia or massive myoclonic seizure
    D. psychomotor epilepsy
    E. none of the above

364. Petit mal (absence attacks) are usually characterized by all of the following EXCEPT
    A. attacks rarely last more than 5 to 15 seconds
    B. typically the child abruptly recovers senses
    C. there is usually no aura
    D. frequency may be increased by fatigue, photic stimulation, and emotional stress
    E. EEG is not characteristic

365. Clinical manifestations of acute postinfectious polyneuritis include all of the following EXCEPT
    A. mild to profound paresis, usually ascending and symmetrical
    B. bilateral facial nerve paresis
    C. paresthesias are common
    D. partial or complete absence of deep tendon reflexes
    E. increased CSF pressure, elevated cell count to 3000 monocytes

366. Infantile myoclonic seizures
    A. have also been called petit mal seizures
    B. usually involve a single muscle group
    C. may recur several hundred times a day
    D. are very difficult to differentiate from pyknolepsy on EEG
    E. are best treated with phenobarbital

367. "Migraine" in children is characterized by
    A. absence of an aura
    B. onset in early childhood
    C. negative family history
    D. unrelated to stress
    E. relief of attack by sleep

DIRECTIONS: Each set of lettered headings below is followed by a list of numbered words or phrases. For each numbered word or phrase select

    A if the item is associated with **A** only,
    B if the item is associated with **B** only,
    C if the item is associated with both **A** and **B**,
    D if the item is associated with neither **A** nor **B**.

    A. Cerebellar astrocytoma
    B. Medulloblastoma
    C. Both
    D. Neither

368. The most common posterior fossa tumor in children

369. Treatment and diagnosis involve surgery

370. Long-term survival is characteristically poor

371. Radiotherapy is not helpful

372. May present with signs of increased intracranial pressure

    A. Subdural hematoma
    B. Extradural hematoma
    C. Both
    D. Neither

373. May exist without skull fracture

374. High incidence in children less than one year of age

375. Subhyaloid hemorrhages occur

376. May occur from venous bleeding

377. The most lethal complication of head injury

    A. Neurofibromatosis
    B. Sturge-Weber syndrome
    C. Both
    D. Neither

378. Autosomal dominant inheritance

379. High incidence of mental retardation

380. Ceroid lipofuscinosis is a common complication

381. Intracranial calcifications are pathognomonic

Table 9 Stages of Reye Syndrome

Stage	Signs and Symptoms
1	Vomiting, lethargy
2	Disorientation, hyperventilation
3	Coma, decorticate posturing, preservation of pupillary light reflexes
4	Deep coma, large fixed pupils, decerebrate posturing, loss of doll's eyes
5	Flaccid paralysis, absent deep DTRs, respiratory arrest

382. Manifestations of the disease involve the skin

    A. Reye syndrome (Table 9)
    B. Viral encephalitis
    C. Both
    D. Neither

383. Associated clotting defects found

384. Personality changes common initial manifestation

385. CSF protein elevated

386. Steroids helpful in improving prognosis

387. Control of increased intracranial pressure essential in therapy

---

DIRECTIONS: Each group of questions below consists of five lettered headings, followed by a list of numbered words, phrases or statements. For each numbered word, phrase or statement, select the **one** lettered heading that is most closely associated with it. Each lettered heading may be selected once, more than once, or not at all.

      A. Bitemporal hemianopsia
      B. Repetitive inappropriate motor acts
      C. Ptosis
      D. Urinary incontinence
      E. Rapid pendular nystagmoid movements

388. Psychomotor seizures

389. Spasmus nutans

390. Craniopharyngioma

391. Juvenile myasthenia gravis

392. Meningomyelocele

DIRECTIONS: This section consists of situations, each followed by a series of questions. Study each situation, and select the **one** best answer to each question following it.

CASE 1 (Questions 393–394): A four and one-half-year-old boy has a four-month history of increasing neurologic disorders. The findings include paresis of conjugate gaze, hemiparesis and hyperreflexia, Babinski response, horizontal nystagmus, and truncal and extremity ataxia. The child does not exhibit sensory defects. Basal ganglia manifestations are not detected. CSF pressure, cell count, protein, and sugar are normal. Plain x-rays of the skull are normal.

393. At this point the diagnosis is probably
   A. Sydenham chorea
   B. meningitis
   C. pinealoma
   D. agenesis of the corpus callosum
   E. none of the above

394. Computerized axial tomography reveals a posterior and upward displacement of the aqueduct of Sylvius and the fourth ventricle. Now the most likely diagnosis is a
   A. brainstem glioma
   B. pinealoma
   C. thalamic tumor
   D. ependymoma
   E. astrocytoma

CASE 2 (Questions 395–396): A 15-year-old boy is in a motorcycle accident in which he is struck by a car. The child sustains a closed head injury and minor orthopedic injuries. The patient remains unconscious for three days, followed by several days of stupor. During the three days of coma he exhibited difficulty with respiration and a convulsion. Cerebral edema is strongly suspected.

395. Which of the following would be of LEAST value in management of the patient during the three days of coma?
    A. CSF studies
    B. IV fluids and electrolyte studies
    C. Endotracheal incubation
    D. Treatment with phenytoin
    E. Dexamethasone therapy

396. The patient is discharged from the hospital after 15 days without medications. The parents are concerned about seizures developing later as a result of the injury. All of the following are correct in counseling EXCEPT
    A. late epilepsy occurs in less than 5% of cases of closed head injuries
    B. seizures may occur; peak incidence occurs at 6 to 18 months after injury
    C. the EEG can be used to accurately predict the chances of epilepsy after the injury
    D. some patients are maintained on medications for at least two years, but no absolute criteria have been established
    E. penetrating depressed fractures have a seizure incidence of 30 to 60% when associated with prolonged unconsciousness

CASE 3 (Questions 397–398): A three-year-old had myoclonic seizures during infancy and later developed grand mal and psychomotor seizures. He was presumed to be mentally retarded, was hyperactive and destructive, and displayed bright red and brown nodules in a butterfly distribution over nose and cheeks. The child died, and autopsy revealed sclerotic patches scattered throughout the gray matter of the cerebral cortex. These patches consisted of astrocytes and bizarre giant cells. Calcium was found in some of the patches. Small tumors made up of fibrous tissue, smooth muscle, and blood vessels were found in the kidney, heart, and liver.

397. The most likely diagnosis in this case is
    A. tuberous sclerosis
    B. malignant glioblastoma
    C. miliary tuberculosis
    D. chronic lymphocytic leukemia
    E. lupus erythematosus

398. Although not described, examination of the eye would probably have revealed
    A. ptosis of the eyelids
    B. cataracts
    C. coarse nystagmus
    D. visual acuity of 20/200
    E. retinal lesions

Nervous System
Answers and Comments

352. E. Conditions A, B, C, and D are usually associated with involuntary sustained spasms of the muscles involving the neck, trunk, and extremities. These spasms may cause abnormal posturing. On the other hand, chorea, which is characterized by sudden, irregular jerking movements is associated with rheumatic fever and can involve any skeletal muscle group including the face. (Ref. 1, p. 1576)

353. B. Postinflammatory or posttraumatic obstruction of the basilar cistern and subarachnoid pathways are the most common causes of hydrocephalus. Fibrosis secondary to intracranial bleeding at birth and meningitis can result in obstruction. (Ref. 1, p. 1591)

354. C. The frequency of occurrence in female fetuses and prematures may be as high as seven times that encountered in males. (Ref. 1, p. 1589)

355. A. Headache in children may not be a reliable nor a localizing sign for brain tumor. Headache may be intermittent, and its frequency is unrelated to site, i.e. infra or supratentorial. (Ref. 1, p. 1622)

356. B. Cerebellar astrocytoma in childhood has a relatively quiet onset and is slowly progressive. The majority of children have symptoms two to seven months before diagnosis. In some cases this latent period may be several years. (Ref. 1, p. 1625)

357. C. Seizures are not common with medulloblastoma. When they do occur they probably represent seeding of the tumor on the cerebral hemispheres. (Ref. 1, p. 1626)

358. E. Diabetes insipidus is an uncommon complication of craniopharyngioma. Other manifestations of hypothalamic dysfunction are more common: growth retardation, obesity, etc. These usually appear postoperatively; somatic and sexual infantilism occur preoperatively. (Ref. 1, p. 1632)

359. A. The changes in gait and posture are caused by weakness, spasticity, and/or an attempt to avoid pain. There is a tendency to avoid flexing at the trunk. Paraspinal muscle spasm occurs; gait disturbances reflect lower extremity involvement and changes in muscle tone. (Ref. 1, p. 1633)

360. B. Pseudotumor cerebri is a syndrome caused by intracranial hypertension. The etiology and pathogenesis are not fully understood. Convulsions and alterations of the mental state do not occur and suggest that the underlying mechanism is unrelated to cerebral edema. (Ref. 1, p. 1636)

361. C. Venous occlusion may be associated with the abscess of the nose. The clinical picture depends on the rapidity and extent of the occlusion. The signs and symptoms presented are compatible with venous thrombosis. (Ref. 1, p. 1638)

362. A. Extradural hemorrhage is not common in children less than two years of age because anatomically the vessels are less adherent to the skull. The hematoma is a result of bleeding between the dura mater and skull. It is often associated with a tear in the middle meningeal artery. (Ref. 1, p. 1647)

363. E. This EEG pattern is believed to arise in the diencephalic nuclei and/or the limbic system. The finding has been detected in a large percentage of clinically normal children. (Ref. 1, p. 1655)

364. E. The EEG in petit mal is very characteristic, usually revealing bursts of generalized bilaterally synchronous three-per-second spike and wave complexes. These occur against a background of relatively normal activity. (Ref. 1, p. 1660)

365. E. The CSF findings are characteristic: pressure is usually normal, cell count is usually normal, sugar is normal, and the protein is elevated. The observation of elevated protein and normal cell count was described by Guillain, Barre, and Strohl. (Ref. 1, p. 1683–1685)

366. C. Infantile myoclonic seizures have also been called "infantile spasms" or "jacknife epilepsy." They occur usually before two years of age and involve more than a single group of muscles.

The EEG changes are characteristic, revealing random high voltage slow waves and spikes. The pattern has been termed hypsarhythmia. The drug of choice is a corticosteroid or pyridoxine. (Ref. 2, p. 1536)

367. E. Migraine is believed to be a common cause of vascular headache in children. A positive family history is found in about two-thirds of patients. The onset is usually in the older child or adolescent. The characteristic aura may include visual disturbances or other transitory neurologic disturbances. Stress increases the number of attacks; sleep relieves the attack. (Ref. 2, p. 1572)

368. B. Both medulloblastoma and cerebellar astrocytoma may
369. C. present with signs of increased intracranial pressure.
370. B. Medulloblastoma is the most common posterior fossa
371. D. tumor and carries a poor prognosis. The DX and RX
372. C. of both tumors requires surgery, and both respond favorably to radiotherapy. (Ref. 1, pp. 1625, 1626)

373. C. Both subdural hematoma and extradural hematoma may
374. A. exist without skull fracture and both can occur from
375. C. venous bleeds. Subhyaloid hemorrhages occur in both
376. C. conditions also. Subdural hematoma is more common
377. B. in children less than one year of age. Extradural hematomas are the most lethal complication of head injury. (Ref. 1, pp. 1647, 1648)

378. A. Both neurofibromatosis and the Sturge-Weber syn-
379. B. drome have skin findings (café-au-lait spots and vascular
380. D. nevi). There is a high incidence of mental retardation
381. B. in the Sturge-Weber syndrome, and the intracranial cal-
382. C. cifications are pathognomonic. Neither syndrome is associated with ceroid lipofuscinosis. (Ref. 1, p. 1763)

383. A. Reye syndrome has associated clotting defects because
384. C. of liver involvement in the disease. Monitoring of in-
385. B. creased intracranial pressure is critical in caring for pa-
386. D. tients with this disease. Viral encephalitis has an
387. A. elevated CSF protein, and like Reye syndrome, presents with bizzare behavior and personality changes. Steroids are not helpful in either disease to improve prognosis. (Ref. 3, p. 86, 585)

388. B. Psychomotor seizures are not usually associated with
389. E. tonic clonic movements, and can be difficult to recognize
390. A. and treat. The EEG may be except during the seizure.
391. C. Spasmus nutans consists of nystagmoid movements with
392. D. head nodding in an otherwise healthy infant in the first two years. Spontaneous improvement is usual, and the etiology is unknown. Because of its frequent occurrence at the optic chiasm, craniopharyngioma frequently presents with progressive visual loss, or signs of increased intracranial pressure. Ptosis is frequently the presenting complaint in myasthenia gravis. Children with meningomyelocele have recurrent urinary tract problems if bladder innervation is affected, in addition to motor defects and hydrocephalus, depending on the location and extent of the malformation. (Ref. 2, pp. 1535, 1561, 1587, 1606, 1754)

393. E. The signs and symptoms described are characteristic of none of the items noted. The neurological findings are most suggestive of brainstem pathology. There is evidence of pyramidal tract and cerebellar pathway involvement, as well as cranial nerve involvement. (Ref. 1, p. 1627)

394. A. The CAT scan in combination with the clinical findings are almost diagnostic of the brainstem glioma. This tumor constitutes 10% of all intracranial tumors in children. (Ref. 1, p. 1627)

395. A. The CSF studies will probably be of little value. The study during the initial acute traumatic period will not be helpful in differentiating extradural, subdural, or intracortical bleeding. Elevated CSF pressure is anticipated. Findings would not determine the course of therapy. (Ref. 1, p. 1648, 1649)

396. C. The EEG is not too reliable a prognostic indicator. Gross irregularity of the EEG after head trauma can be found in a normal child. A normal EEG tends to make posttraumatic epilepsy less likely. A worsening EEG makes one suspicious. The EEG may be a misleading laboratory method of predicting epilepsy posttrauma. (Ref. 1, p. 1650)

397. A. The diagnosis of tuberous sclerosis is strongly suggested by the combined clinical signs. The seizures, retardation, destructive behaviors, and aggressiveness are common as is the changing pattern of seizures characteristic. Skin lesions (adenoma sebaceum) are found in 80% of patients. Confirmation is made by the description of the pathologic lesions. (Ref. 2, p. 1574)

398. E. The characteristic lesions in about half the patients are retinal. They appear as elevated yellow or white areas usually near the edge of the optic disc. The lesions are malformations of the nerve fiber layer of the retina, and as a rule do not impair visual acuity. (Ref. 2, p. 1574)

14 Respiratory System

399. Which of the following is the primary presenting complaint with foreign bodies in the nasal passages?
     A. Pain
     B. Bleeding from the nostril
     C. Watery discharge
     D. Ipsilateral "watery" eye
     E. Obstruction

400. All of the following infectious agents may cause primary acute tonsillopharyngitis EXCEPT
     A. staphylococci
     B. streptococci
     C. viral agents
     D. diphtheria organisms
     E. *Neisseria gonorrhoeae*

157

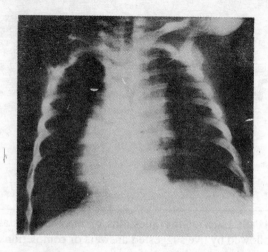

Figure 9 Note the hyperinfection typically found in patients with bronchiolitis.

401. The principal single cause of bronchiolitis (Fig. 9) is
   A. *H. influenzae*
   B. pneumococcus
   C. parainfluenza
   D. Coxsackie A
   E. respiratory syncytial virus

402. The principal single cause of croup syndrome is
   A. *H. influenzae*
   B. respiratory syncytial virus
   C. Coxsackie B
   D. parainfluenza virus
   E. group A streptococci

403. The most common complication of acute nasopharyngitis in children is
   A. bronchitis
   B. sinusitis
   C. otitis media
   D. laryngitis
   E. pneumonia

404. The percentage of normal children who carry streptococci in their throat is
   A. 1% to 2%
   B. 5% to 10%
   C. 15% to 20%
   D. 20% to 25%
   E. 30% to 35%

405. Pharyngitis with conjunctivitis is most often caused by
   A. adenovirus
   B. Coxsackie virus
   C. *H. influenzae*
   D. group A strep
   E. *S. aureus*

406. The most common cause of retropharyngeal abscess is
   A. a penetrating injury of posterior pharyngeal wall
   B. dissection of purulent material from tonsil
   C. suppuration of draining nodes of retropharyngeal spaces
   D. tonsil and adenoid surgery
   E. meningitis

407. Sinobronchitis may be seen in association with all of the following EXCEPT
   A. chronic sinusitis
   B. cystic fibrosis
   C. α-1-antitrypsin deficiency
   D. patients who have allergy and smoke
   E. chronic use of vasoconstrictive nose drops for vaso-motor rhinitis

408. Which of the following statements concerning juvenile papilloma is FALSE?
   A. It is the most common benign tumor of the larynx in children
   B. It usually grows from the vocal cords
   C. It often disappears after age 12 years
   D. The first symptom is hoarseness
   E. It usually disappears by age four years

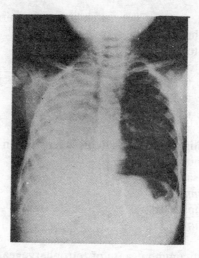

Figure 10 Collapse of the lung due to a foreign body.

409. All of the following may be associated with bronchial foreign bodies (Fig. 10) EXCEPT
  A. differences in valvular mechanisms are responsible in large part for the clinical symptoms
  B. fluoroscopic examination is very valuable as a diagnostic aid
  C. a high percentage of foreign bodies will be spontaneously removed by coughing
  D. secondary infection may occur if removal is delayed
  E. direct visualization by bronchoscopy and removal are commonly employed

410. Infectious croup may be associated with all of the following EXCEPT
  A. parainfluenza virus
  B. *H. influenzae*
  C. a family history of croup in 15% of cases, and a history of recurrent laryngitis in the patient
  D. airway obstruction severe enough to require assisted ventilation
  E. permanent loss of hearing

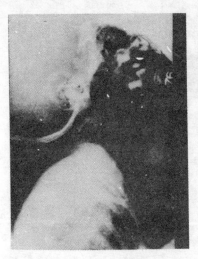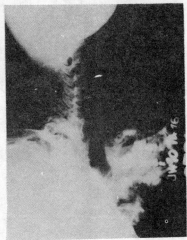

Figure 11 Epiglottitis (*left*) on the lateral neck with normal (*right*) for comparison.

411. In contrast to acute epiglottitis, acute laryngotracheobronchitis (Fig. 11) has all of the following features EXCEPT
    A. a more insidious onset
    B. the etiologic agent is almost always viral
    C. a slower course
    D. the etiologic agent is almost always bacterial
    E. the patient is less likely to require intubation

412. Which of the following would NOT be included in the differential diagnosis of acute infectious croup?
    A. Diphtheria
    B. Foreign body inhalation
    C. Parainfluenza viral infection
    D. Retropharyngeal abscess
    E. Laryngeal papilloma

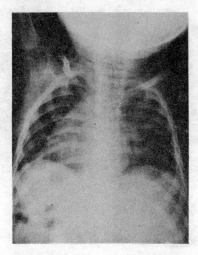

Figure 12 An example of poor inspiration, which can mimic the appearance of pneumonia, especially in young infants.

413. Pneumococcal pneumonia (Fig. 12) is associated with all of the following EXCEPT
   A. it is the most common form of bacterial pneumonia in children
   B. serotypes causing the disease in children differ from those of adults
   C. type specific antibody will provide protection from reinfection
   D. prevention by pneumococcal; vaccine may be possible in older children
   E. sickle cell anemia patients have no demonstrated increased risk factor for this infection, as they do for *Salmonella* infections

414. Concerning the symptoms of pneumococcal pneumonia in childhood, all of the following are true EXCEPT
   A. infants may be free of rales early in the course
   B. meningismus is not uncommon
   C. classic symptoms of consolidation are noted on either the second or third day of the illness
   D. most patients do not give a history of URI
   E. pneumococcal vaccine may not prove to serve as effective prophylaxis in infants under one year of age

415. Kartagener syndrome includes all of the following EXCEPT
  A. occurrence in older patients
  B. presence of complete situs inversus
  C. paranasal sinusitis and bronchiectasis are present
  D. it is a treatable condition, in part
  E. it is often apparent in the first year of life

DIRECTIONS: For each of the questions or incomplete statements below, **one or more** of the answers or completions given is correct. Select

  A   if only **1**, **2**, and **3** are correct,
  B   if only **1** and **3** are correct,
  C   if only **2** and **4** are correct,
  D   if only **4** is correct,
  E   if all are correct.

---

416. Stridor in the newborn may be caused by
  1. laryngomalacia
  2. laryngeal web
  3. laryngeal paralysis secondary to trauma
  4. laryngeal papillomas

417. In patients with cystic fibrosis
  1. there is always a positive family history
  2. the earliest pulmonary symptoms may be coughing
  3. bronchopleural fistulas are common
  4. cor pulmonale may develop

418. Diseases that mainly affect the pulmonary interstitium include
  1. sarcoidosis
  2. hypersensitivity lung disease
  3. pulmonary hemosiderosis
  4. systemic lupus erythematous with pulmonary involvement

Directions Summarized				
A	B	C	D	E
1,2,3	1,3	2,4	4	All are
only	only	only	only	correct

419. In regard to familial pectus excavatum
1. it is a common feature in congenital heart disease
2. surgical repair is indicated
3. lung capacity is usually decreased by 15%
4. it is rarely, if ever, a cause of pulmonary disability

420. Indications for tonsillectomy include
1. frequent respiratory infections
2. symptomatic hypertrophy with signs and symptoms of obstruction
3. chronic otitis media
4. chronic tonsillar infection

421. In congenital diaphragmatic hernia
1. the diagnosis may be suggested by auscultating bowel sounds in the thorax
2. pulmonary hypoplasia is common
3. surgery is indicated
4. mechanical ventilation has not increased survival

DIRECTIONS: This section consists of situations, each followed by a series of questions. Study each situation, and select the **one** best answer to each question following it.

CASE 1 (Questions 422–426): You are asked to consult on a case of failure to thrive in a six-month-old girl. There is a history of bulky diarrheal stools, and chronic cough. Your initial suspicion from history alone is that cystic fibrosis is an important diagnostic consideration.

422. True statements about this disease include all of the following EXCEPT
   A. prognosis is steadily improving with up to 50% cumulative survival rate
   B. pulmonary infection causes most of the morbidity
   C. it is inherited as a sex-linked recessive disease
   D. administration of influenza vaccine is indicated in these patients
   E. the basic defect remains unknown

423. Complications of the disease include all of the following EXCEPT
   A. meconium ileus
   B. hypoglycemic episodes
   C. rectal prolapse
   D. nasal polyps
   E. biliary cirrhosis

424. Infections of the respiratory tract commonly seen in patients with cystic fibrosis include each of the following EXCEPT
   A. *Pseudomonas*
   B. *Staphylococcus aureus*
   C. pneumococcus
   D. *Pneumocystis carinii*
   E. *Aspergillus*

425. Pulmonary complications of the disease include all of the following EXCEPT
    A. pneumothorax
    B. atelectasis
    C. hemoptysis
    D. acute respiratory failure
    E. pleuritis

426. Treatment of this disease should include
    A. genetic counseling for the parents
    B. pancreatic enzymes given once a day
    C. corticosteroids to reduce pulmonary inflammation in most patients
    D. iodides and glycerol guaiacolate to improve expectoration
    E. long-term bronchodilator therapy

Respiratory System
Answers and Comments

399. E. Obstruction may well be followed by malodorous purulent discharge. (Ref. 2, p. 1012)

400. A. Staphylococcal organisms may be recovered by culture, but do not cause primary disease in this location. (Ref. 2, p. 1015)

401. E. RSV is the most important respiratory tract pathogen found in the first two to three years of life. (Ref. 2, p. 1044)

402. D. Parainfluenza virus causes the majority of cases of croup syndrome, and is also a cause of bronchitis and URI. (Ref. 2, p. 1034)

403. C. Otitis media occurs most commonly in infants and can be expected if fever recurs. (Ref. 2, p. 1025)

404. C. This high percentage of carriers may make diagnosis in sick children difficult. (Ref. 2, p. 633)

405. A. In adenoviral pharyngitis, the most striking finding is follicular injection of bulbar and palpebral conjunctiva. (Ref. 2, p. 782)

406. C. These nodes drain portions of the nasopharynx and posterior nasal passages. (Ref. 2, p. 1017)

407. E. The use of vasoconstrictor nose drops may well cause rebound rhinitis but it is not a known etiology for the sinobronchitis syndrome. (Ref. 2, p. 1019)

408. E. There is a high rate of recurrence with these lesions after surgical removal. Often after age 12 years, the lesions do not recur. (Ref. 2, p. 1041)

409. C. Only 2 to 4% of foreign bodies are coughed up. (Ref. 2, p. 1038)

410. E. All of the statements are true concerning infectious croup except permanent hearing loss, which has not been described. (Ref. 2, p. 1034)

411. D. All of the statements concerning laryngotracheobronchitis are true except D. The etiologic agent is usually viral and contrasts vividly with epiglottitis, which is usually a rapidly progressing *Haemophilus* infection with abrupt onset. (Ref. 2, p. 1035)

412. E. With benefit of adequate history, laryngeal papilloma would not be included because of the presence of hoarseness weeks before airway obstruction becomes a problem. All of the other etiologies are possibilities, with viral etiology the most common. (Ref. 2, p. 1034)

413. E. All of the statements are true except E. Sickle cell anemia patients are at increased risk for pneumococcal infection. (Ref. 2, p. 1048)

414. D. Most patients do describe a brief upper respiratory infection. (Ref. 2, p. 1048)

415. E. This is a symptom complex seen only in older patients. (Ref. 2, p. 1043)

416. E. All of the choices listed can be the cause of stridor in the newborn infant. (Ref. 1, p. 913)

417. C. The earliest symptom of cystic fibrosis may be cough. Cor pulmonale is a late finding, after pulmonary fibrosis has occurred and pulmonary hypertension has become severe. Bronchopleural fistulae are rare complications. Most cases of CF are sporadic, representing spontaneous mutations. (Ref. 1, p. 1434–1436)

418. E. All of the items listed involve pulmonary interstitium. (Ref. 1, p. 1448–1450)

419. D. Pectus excavatum is rarely, if ever, a cause of pulmonary disability nor is it a common feature of CHD. Surgery is not indicated. (Ref. 1, p. 1454)

420. C. Of those listed, the only indications for tonsillectomy are symptomatic hypertrophy and chronically infected tonsils. (Ref. 2, p. 1020)

421. A. In congenital diaphragmatic hernia the diagnosis may be suggested by auscultating bowel sounds in the chest. Surgery is absolutely indicated, and mechanical ventilation increases the chances of survival tremendously. Pulmonary hypoplasia is common. (Ref. 1, p. 1388)

422. C. Cystic fibrosis is an autosomal recessive disease whose
423. B. basic defect remains unknown. Most of the morbidity
424. D. comes from pulmonary involvement, with a wide variety
425. E. of chronic infections and complications possible. Me-
426. A. conium ileus, the most common cause of intestinal obstruction in the newborn, allows immediate diagnosis in about 10% of patients. Rectal prolapse, nasal polyps, and biliary cirrhosis may be associated features of the disease. None of the treatments in question 426 are appropriate except genetic counseling of the parents. With improving methods for control of pulmonary disease, the survival rate continues to improve. (Ref. 3, p. 215)

15 Gastrointestinal System

DIRECTIONS: Each of the questions or incomplete statements below is followed by five suggested answers or completions. Select the **one** that is best in each case.

---

427. A flat postabsorptive blood sugar curve can be observed in diarrheal states because of all of the following EXCEPT
    A. defects of absorption
    B. increased gut motility
    C. delayed gastric emptying
    D. defects of digestion
    E. disturbance of renal function

171

```
COMPOSITION OF WORLD HEALTH ORGANIZATION

ORAL REHYDRATION SOLUTION (mM/l)

Na              90
K               20
Cl              80
HCO3            30
glucose         111
osmolality      331
```

Figure 13 Composite of WHO oral rehydration solution.

428. The minimal fluid intake recommended for a six-month-old
     infant with mild diarrhea (Fig. 13) is
     A. 300 ml/kg/24 hr
     B. 75 ml/kg/24 hr
     C. 150 ml/kg/24 hr
     D. 50 ml/kg/24 hr
     E. 500 ml/kg/24 hr

429. Which is NOT a common finding in the patient with glucose-
     galactose malabsorption?
     A. Normal intestinal disaccharide activity
     B. Glycosuria
     C. Severe, watery diarrhea on ingestion of glucose
     D. Constipation
     E. Severe, watery diarrhea with milk ingestion

430. The most definitive method of diagnosing disaccharide mal-
     absorption is
     A. family history
     B. biopsy and direct assay
     C. tolerance tests utilizing blood sugar assay
     D. stool pH
     E. reducing substances positive in the stool

431. Protein-losing gastroenteropathy has been associated with
     all of the following EXCEPT
     A. cow milk protein
     B. lymphangiectasia
     C. granulomatous disease of the intestine
     D. ulcerative colitis
     E. soy protein formula

432. Which of the following statements regarding the stools of a child with irritable colon syndrome is FALSE?
   A. They number three to 10 per day
   B. They usually are passed in the space of a few hours early in the day
   C. They often contain mucus
   D. They frequently are bloody
   E. They may contain particles of undigested food, such as corn kernels

433. Irritable colon syndrome in children is associated with
   A. steatorrhea
   B. protein malabsorption
   C. growth failure
   D. pathogenic bacteria in the stools
   E. spontaneous remissions

434. The treatment for irritable colon syndrome in a two-year-old is
   A. low-fat diet
   B. milk-free diet
   C. low-residue diet
   D. low-carbohydrate diet
   E. normal diet for age

435. Organic causes for the symptom of chronic abdominal pain include all of the following EXCEPT
   A. constipation
   B. regional enteritis
   C. urinary tract infection
   D. chronic appendicitis
   E. ulcerative colitis

436. The major organic cause for recurrent abdominal pain in children is
   A. peptic ulcer
   B. regional enteritis
   C. Meckel's diverticulum
   D. urinary tract disease
   E. Hirschsprung disease

Table 10 Study the Accompanying Illustration

Feature	Hirschsprung Disease	Acquired Megacolon
History		
From birth	Always	Never
Enterocolitis	Possible	None
Coercive bowel training	Absent	Usually present
Encopresis	Never	Always
Size of stool	Normal small	Huge
Examination		
Abdominal distension	Possible	Absent
Anal tone	Tight	Patulous
Feces in ampulla	Never	Packed with stool

437. The most useful clinical tool for differentiating congenital
aganglionosis from functional constipation (Table 10) is
A. early onset of symptoms
B. marked infrequency of stools
C. appearance of stools
D. absence of the urge to defecate
E. response to laxative therapy

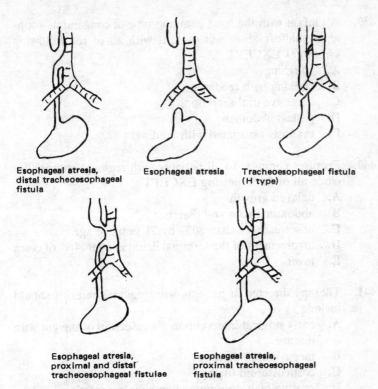

Esophageal atresia,
distal tracheoesophageal
fistula

Esophageal atresia

Tracheoesophageal fistula
(H type)

Esophageal atresia,
proximal and distal
tracheoesophageal fistulae

Esophageal atresia,
proximal tracheoesophageal
fistula

Figure 14 Anatomy of major types of tracheoesophageal malformations in newborns.

438. The most common type of congenital esophageal malformation (Fig. 14) is
   A. esophageal atresia with distal tracheoesophageal fistula
   B. esophageal atresia without fistula
   C. tracheoesophageal fistula without atresia
   D. esophageal atresia with proximal tracheoesophageal fistula
   E. esophageal atresia, and proximal and distal tracheoesophageal fistula

439. An infant with the most common type of congenital esophageal malformation will present with all of the following symptoms EXCEPT
A. coughing
B. choking with feedings
C. excessive oral secretions
D. gasless abdomen
E. cyanosis associated with feedings

440. Features common to all patients with regional enteritis include all of the following EXCEPT
A. delayed growth
B. abdominal pain and diarrhea
C. onset in more than 80% by 21 years of age
D. involvement of the terminal ileum in over 80% of cases
E. fever

441. Therapy directed at patients with regional enteritis should include
A. early surgical intervention via resection of the gut with disease
B. megavitamin therapy
C. corticosteroid therapy
D. routine high-dose potassium supplementation
E. high-fiber diet

442. Which of the following features is NOT part of the clinical course in the patient with ulcerative colitis?
A. Diarrhea and abdominal pain are the most common presenting features
B. Barium enema is always diagnostic at the onset of symptoms
C. Anemia is common
D. Liver disease is an uncommon complication in children
E. Colectomy

443. All of the following are true concerning intussusception EXCEPT
  A. it usually affects infants in the first two years of life
  B. a local lesion is usually found as a cause
  C. most cases begin at or near the ileocecal valve
  D. males are more frequently affected than females
  E. a stool mixed with blood and mucus is often passed

444. The signs and symptoms of intussusception may include all of the following EXCEPT
  A. the infant is well nourished and hydrated
  B. attacks of colicky pain recurring regularly with intervals in which the infant is in no distress
  C. the presence of blood and mucus in the stools
  D. vomiting rarely occurs as an initial symptom
  E. abdominal pain is a frequent presenting complaint

445. Which of the following statements is true in regard to the treatment of intussusception?
  A. Treatment should be delayed for four to six hours owing to the high incidence of spontaneous reduction
  B. Recurrence is more common after hydrostatic pressure reduction than operative reduction
  C. Hydrostatic pressure reduction is the method of choice
  D. Distension is an absolute contraindication for hydrostatic pressure reduction
  E. Rupture of bowel is frequently a complication of hydrostatic pressure reduction

446. Rectal prolapse can be seen in children with all of the following EXCEPT
  A. cystic fibrosis
  B. severe malnutrition
  C. whooping cough
  D. phimosis
  E. pinworm infestation

447. Concerning benign polyps of the GI tract, which of the following is FALSE?
   A. Most common intestinal tumor
   B. Usually occurs in the colon
   C. Most frequent symptom is bleeding
   D. Bleeding is usually profuse
   E. Blood is generally bright red

448. Which of the following is FALSE concerning lymphosarcoma of the bowel in childhood?
   A. Most common malignant tumor of the bowel
   B. Terminal ileum is most common site
   C. Usually diagnosed early because of intestinal obstruction
   D. Bleeding is rare
   E. History of chronic intussusception may be obtained

449. All of the following metabolic alterations can occur in pyloric stenosis EXCEPT
   A. hypokalemia
   B. hypochloremia
   C. decreased serum pH
   D. dehydration
   E. alkalosis

450. All of the following may be features of pyloric stenosis EXCEPT
   A. it is more common in males
   B. it usually becomes symptomatic in the first month of life
   C. initially there is nonprojectile vomiting
   D. vomitus is bile stained
   E. failure to thrive

451. Which of the following statements concerning congenital high intestinal obstructions is FALSE?
   A. Vomiting may be persistent if there is no feeding of the infant
   B. Polyhydramnios is a frequent accompaniment
   C. Meconium stools may be passed initially
   D. Vomitus is always bile stained
   E. Farber test has limited value

452. All of the following statements are true of intestinal occlusions present at birth EXCEPT
   A. stenosis is more common than atresia
   B. the ileum is the site of 50% of the lesions
   C. infants with Down syndrome have an increased incidence of duodenal atresia
   D. in about 15% of infants, multiple intestinal occlusions occur
   E. symptoms may or may not be present at birth

453. All of the following are true concerning Meckel's diverticulum EXCEPT
   A. it occurs in 2 to 3% of all persons
   B. mucosal lining may be gastric, and this is the type most likely to produce symptoms
   C. symptoms most commonly occur in the first two years of life
   D. mucosal lining may be gastric and ileal, or colonic and ileal
   E. acute painful hemorrhage is the most common symptom

454. The absence of ganglion cells of the intramural and submucous plexuses of the colon may be manifest by all of the following EXCEPT
   A. severe enterocolitis in the neonate
   B. the lesion occurs in 90% of cases in an area of bowel 4 to 25 cm proximal to the anus
   C. a patient who fails to thrive
   D. history of obstipation and abdominal distension from early infancy
   E. large stools and fecal soiling are common symptoms in children more than 5 years of age

455. Australia antigen is a marker associated with
   A. infectious hepatitis
   B. serum hepatitis
   C. hepatitis of any viral etiology
   D. alcoholic hepatitis
   E. α 1-antitrypsin deficiency

456. All of the following are symptoms characteristic of the early
     phase of infectious hepatitis EXCEPT
     A. fever
     B. malaise
     C. anorexia
     D. jaundice
     E. nausea and vomiting

457. Which of the major nutrients is less likely to have decreased
     absorption during diarrhea?
     A. Fat
     B. Monosaccharides
     C. Protein
     D. Starch
     E. Disaccharides

DIRECTIONS: Each group of questions below consists of five
lettered headings followed by a list of numbered words, phrases,
or statements. For each numbered word, phrase, or statement,
select the **one** lettered heading that is most closely associated with
it. Each lettered heading may be selected once, more than once,
or not at all.

     A. Esophageal atresia
     B. Pyloric stenosis
     C. Chalasia
     D. Duodenal atresia
     E. Intussusception

458. High incidence in Down syndrome

459. Bloody stool may be seen

460. Surgery is usually not indicated

461. Passage of radiopaque catheter is usually diagnostic

462. More frequent in male infants

463. Barium enema is indicated if there is no intestinal
     perforation

DIRECTIONS: This section consists of situations, each followed by a series of questions. Study each situation and select the **one** best answer to the questions following it.

CASE 1 (Questions 464–466): An eight-month-old infant is referred to you for failure to thrive and chronic diarrhea. There is a family history of celiac disease. You consult your texts to familiarize yourself with this disease, and plan a work-up (Fig. 15).

Figure 15 Physical growth for age, boys: birth to 36 months.

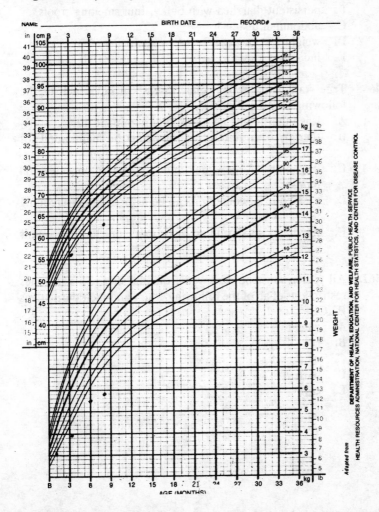

464. Differential diagnosis at this point may include each of the following EXCEPT
- **A.** secondary disaccharidase deficiency
- **B.** cystic fibrosis
- **C.** cow's milk protein sensitivity
- **D.** celiac sprue
- **E.** chronic nonspecific diarrhea of infancy

465. Clinical manifestations of celiac disease include all of the following EXCEPT
- **A.** unresponsive iron deficiency
- **B.** persistent diarrhea with bulky, foul smelling stools
- **C.** abdominal distension
- **D.** weight loss or poor growth velocity
- **E.** increased appetite

466. True statements about celiac disease include each of the following EXCEPT
- **A.** it is inherited as an autosomal dominant trait
- **B.** therapy of a gluten-free diet must be maintained for life
- **C.** flattening of intestinal villi are noted on intestinal biopsy
- **D.** a 72-hour fat collection can be a good initial screening test
- **E.** the diagnosis should never be made on clinical grounds alone

467. All gluten must be removed from the diet. This includes restrictions of all of the following grains and their derivatives EXCEPT
- **A.** wheat
- **B.** rye
- **C.** oats
- **D.** barley
- **E.** corn

468. True statements about the treatment of this condition include all of the following EXCEPT
    A. oral iron may be indicated
    B. fat soluble vitamins K and D may need to be supplemented initially
    C. steroids frequently aid in more rapid resolution of the disease
    D. resolution of symptoms occurs within weeks, with improvement in irritability within days
    E. within six months patients are frequently within the normal range for weight

Gastrointestinal System
Answers and Comments

427. E. All of these factors except renal excretion defects would influence postprandial blood sugar curves. The only accurate method of measuring carbohydrate absorption is radioactive labeling. (Ref. 1, p. 924)

428. C. The minimum amount is 150 ml/kg/24 hr, and 300 ml/kg/24 hr would be unusual. (Ref. 1, p. 924)

429. D. Glycosuria is a common finding. Acquired malabsorption has been described in patients with surgical resections and acute episodes of gastroenteritis. Milk causes diarrhea because intestinal lactase breaks milk sugar down into glucose and galactose. (Ref. 1, p. 936)

430. B. Biopsy of mucosa of small intestine and direct assay of disaccharides are the most definitive methods. (Ref. 1, pp. 1004, 1005, 935)

431. E. These children will suffer from edema and will demonstrate hypoproteinemia without proteinuria. Protein-losing gastroenteropathy has not been described in association with soy protein ingestion. (Ref. 1, p. 936)

432. D. This syndrome usually begins at about 6 months and ceases between 3 or 4 years of age. Blood is not detectable in the stool. (Ref. 1, p. 937)

433. E. These children grow normally despite recurrent bouts of loose stools. Spontaneous remissions at age three to four years are the rule. (Ref. 1, p. 938)

434. E. Dietary modifications are unnecessary, are potentially harmful, and lead to nutritionally unbalanced diets and unnecessary parental concern. Some advocate avoidance of iced foods for children with this syndrome. (Ref. 1, p. 938)

435. D.   Chronic appendicitis, and chronic mesenteric lymphadenitis are diagnoses in considerable doubt in modern pediatrics. (Ref. 1, p. 941)

436. D.   Every patient with the complaint of recurrent abdominal pain deserves urinalysis. (Ref. 1, p. 941)

437. D.   The proprioceptors that initiate the reflex urge to defecate are located just proximal to the internal sphincter and are rarely activated in the patient with Hirschsprung disease. (Ref. 1, p. 943)

438. A.   This variety accounts for about 86% of all cases. (Ref. 1, p. 946)

439. D.   The distal tracheoesophageal fistula allows large quantities of air into the gastrointestinal tract. (Ref. 1, p. 945)

440. C.   Onset of illness has been reported to be 10 to 15% by age 15 years; about half experience onset by 21 years. (Ref. 1, p. 979)

441. C.   Corticosteroid therapy is eventually required for most patients and is useful in control of the disease. Mega-vitamin therapy is of no proved benefit. Surgical intervention is restricted to specific complications. (Ref. 1, p. 980)

442. B.   Barium enema may appear entirely normal for periods of up to two to three years after onset of disease. (Ref. 1, p. 981, 982)

443. B.   A cause is rarely clear. In only 2.5% of cases under two years of age is a cause identifiable. (Ref. 1, p. 989)

444. D.   Abdominal pain and vomiting are common initial symptoms. (Ref. 1, p. 989)

445. C.   Hydrostatic pressure reduction is the method of choice because discomfort is less than with surgery. The complications in the absence of anesthesia are fewer, and the period of hospitalization is much shorter. (Ref. 1, p. 989)

446. E. All of these conditions except pinworms have been associated with rectal prolapse. Recurrent episodes are most commonly seen with patients with cystic fibrosis. Any condition that increases the intraabdominal pressure may precipitate prolapse, and malnutrition may be a significant contributing factor. (Ref. 1, p. 990)

447. D. Rarely is bleeding from benign polyps profuse. The blood may be mixed with the stool or be present on the surface of the stool. (Ref. 1, p. 992)

448. C. The tumor is usually discovered quite late owing to its insidious infiltration, which eventually leads to intestinal obstruction. (Ref. 1, p. 992)

449. C. Pyloric stenosis usually results in hypochloremic alkalosis. This can be corrected by the administration of fluids containing sodium and potassium. (Ref. 2, p. 242)

450. D. The vomitus is not bile stained in pyloric stenosis. (Ref. 2, p. 904)

451. D. The vomitus will contain bile if the obstruction is below the ampulla of Vater as is usually, but not always, the case. (Ref. 2, p. 906)

452. A. Atresia is the more common lesion. Symptoms may be delayed an indeterminate length of time if the obstruction is incomplete. (Ref. 2, p. 906)

453. E. Bleeding is the most common symptom, but it is not accompanied by pain. Bleeding is usually acute, but may be intermittent and recurrent. (Ref. 2, p. 912)

454. E. The stools of the older infant or child may have a consistency of small pellets or be ribbon-like or have a fluid consistency. Large stools and fecal soiling are typical of the patient with functional consipation. (Ref. 2, p. 910)

455. B. Serum, or long incubation type B hepatitis frequently contains this antigen. (Ref. 2, p. 784)

456. D. All the other symptoms usually occur four to five days before the onset of jaundice. (Ref. 2, p. 786)

457. C. Protein assimilation is affected relatively little. (Ref. 1, p. 924)

458. D. The diagnosis of intussusception is confirmed by barium
459. E. enema, and this procedure can be curative, and is in-
460. C. dicated if perforation has not occurred. Bloody stool is
461. A. common. There is a high incidence of duodenal atresia
462. B. in Down syndrome. Chalasia is not considered a surgical
463. E. problem. Pyloric stenosis is seen more commonly in males. Esophageal atresia can be diagnosed by the passage of a radiopaque catheter. (Ref. 2, pp. 904–914)

464. E. All of the conditions listed would be considered in the
465. E. differential in this case, except chronic nonspecific diar-
466. A. rhea of infancy, which does not cause failure to thrive.
467. E. Decreased appetite is more a feature of the disease than
468. C. increased appetite. All of the other clinical manifestations given are characteristic. The mode of genetic transmission is undetermined. It is essential that the diagnosis be confirmed by biopsy, since therapeutic diet is life long! All of the grains listed, except corn, should be eliminated. Steroids have no place in the therapy of this disease. (Ref. 3, p. 221 and Ref. 2, p. 933)

16 Blood and Blood-Forming Tissues

DIRECTIONS: Each of the questions or incomplete statements below is followed by five suggested answers or completions. Select the **one** that is best in each case.

---

469. In which of the following organs is erythropoietin primarily produced?
    A. Bone marrow
    B. Liver
    C. Kidney
    D. Spleen
    E. Intestines

470. Which of the following globin chain combinations is present in hemoglobin F?
    A. Alpha 2 gamma 2
    B. Alpha 2 beta 2
    C. Alpha 2 delta 2
    D. Alpha 2 epsilon 2
    E. Epsilon 4

471. Which of the following approximates the blood volume in older children?
   A. 90 ml/kg
   B. 85 ml/kg
   C. 80 ml/kg
   D. 75 ml/kg
   E. 70 ml/kg

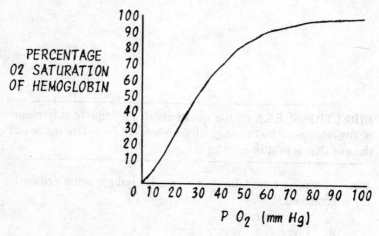

PERCENTAGE O2 SATURATION OF HEMOGLOBIN

P O$_2$ (mm Hg)

Figure 16 Oxygen hemoglobin dissociation curve.

472. A shift of the oxygen dissociation curve (Fig. 16) to the right (decreased affinity of the RBC for oxygen) is associated with all of the following EXCEPT
   A. high altitude
   B. cyanosis
   C. anemia
   D. fetal life
   E. none of the above

473. A low mean corpuscular volume (MCV) in the face of anemia is associated with which one of the following?
   A. Thalassemia minor
   B. Reticulocytosis
   C. Liver disease
   D. Chronic hypoplastic anemia
   E. Folate deficiency

474. A normal MCV and a normal reticulocyte index is usually associated with which one of the following?
   A. Chronic disease
   B. Malignancy with bone marrow involvement
   C. Acute blood loss
   D. Acute aplastic anemia
   E. Malignancy without bone marrow involvement

475. Abnormalities associated with intravascular hemolysis include all of the following EXCEPT
   A. increase in plasma hemoglobin
   B. decrease in serum haptoglobin
   C. increase in urinary hemosiderin
   D. increase in serum unconjugated bilirubin
   E. none of the above

476. Under which one of the following circumstances is iron absorption in the small intestine decreased?
   A. When it is complexed with fructose
   B. When it is complexed with ascorbic acid
   C. When it is complexed with histidine
   D. When it is complexed with lysine
   E. By formation of insoluble phosphates

477. With which one of the following is a depressed serum ferritin (less than 7 mg/ml) more often associated?
   A. Chronic renal disease
   B. Rheumatoid arthritis
   C. Iron deficiency anemia
   D. Infection
   E. Malignancy

478. Which one of the following is the single most useful aid to early diagnosis of folate deficiency?
   A. RBC indicies
   B. Serum folate
   C. Hypersegmentation of neutrophil nuclei
   D. Bone marrow aspiration
   E. Whole blood folate

479. Juvenile pernicious anemia is characterized by all of the following EXCEPT
  A. gastric atrophy
  B. concurrent abnormalities
  C. selective IgA deficiency
  D. autosomal recessive inheritance pattern
  E. chronic candidiasis

480. Which one of the following is the earliest clinical manifestation of vitamin B_{12} deficiency?
  A. Hypersegmented neutrophils
  B. Megaloblastic anemia
  C. Thrombocytopenia
  D. Mild jaundice
  E. Leukopenia

481. Anemia of infection and chronic disease is associated with all of the following EXCEPT
  A. shortened red cell survival
  B. impaired utilization of iron
  C. normal amount of iron in erythroid precursors
  D. impaired erythropoietin and marrow response
  E. usually mild anemia with normocytic or microcytic red cells

482. Acquired aplastic anemia is commonly associated with all of the following EXCEPT
  A. hepatosplenomegaly
  B. purpura
  C. no characteristic morphologic abnormalities are evident on peripheral blood smear
  D. increase in the iron saturation of serum transferrin
  E. absence of adenopathy

483. Congenital aplastic anemia is commonly associated with all of the following EXCEPT
   A. hematologic manifestations appear after five years of age
   B. peripheral blood that reveals a macrocytic, normo-chromic anemia
   C. skeletal malformations of the upper extremities
   D. leukemia
   E. anemia is the usual presenting picture

484. Anti-D antibody (RhoGAM) should be administered to mothers under all the following circumstances EXCEPT
   A. Rh-negative mother not previously sensitized deliver-ing a Rh-positive infant
   B. Rh-negative mother whose pregnancy has been ter-minated by an abortion
   C. mothers tested as Rh-negative whose red cells contain the D^u allele
   D. Rh-negative mothers who deliver infants who are D^u antigen-positive
   E. Rh-negative mother who has had an abortion prior to delivering an Rh-positive infant

485. Erythroblastosis fetalis is associated with all of the following EXCEPT
   A. fetal response to anemia with increased release of eryth-ropoietin and increased hematopoiesis
   B. hepatic cellular necrosis in severe disease
   C. hypoinsulinism
   D. fetal growth is usually normal
   E. appearance of pulmonary surfactant is low

486. Which of the following is FALSE concerning drug-induced hemolytic anemia?
  A. Drugs are rarely the cause of hemolysis in children
  B. A positive Coombs' test may be found in patients receiving penicillin in high doses
  C. Cephalothin commonly acts as an hapten, and in the ensuing reaction, hemolytic anemia may develop
  D. Alpha-methyldopa is the most common cause of drug-induced hemolytic anemia
  E. The antibody formed against the combination of red cell membrane and penicillin is IgG

487. Paroxysmal nocturnal hemoglobinuria is characterized by all of the following EXCEPT
  A. it is associated with a low plasma pH
  B. other elements of the blood (WBC and platelets) are usually normal
  C. major thrombotic episodes occasionally occur
  D. the disease may terminate in leukemia
  E. intravascular hemolysis

488. Which of the following statements is FALSE regarding the pathophysiology of sickle cell disease?
  A. Infection is associated with increased anemia by suppression of RBC production
  B. Conversion of RBC from normal biconcave discs to sickle forms require the deoxygenation of hemoglobin
  C. Hypoxia and acidemia promote sickling by decreasing oxygen saturation of hemoglobin
  D. Dehydration does not promote sickling
  E. Sickle cells increase whole blood viscosity, producing local ischemia

489. Which one of the following clinical manifestations is NOT common to sickle cell disease?
   A. Vasoocclusive crisis is more common than aplastic crisis
   B. Hyperhemolytic crisis is often associated with red cell G6PD deficiency
   C. Aplastic crisis is often associated with viral or bacterial infection
   D. Salmonella sepsis is commonly associated with Salmonella osteomyelitis
   E. Hand–foot syndrome may be the initial manifestation of sickle cell disease

490. Sickle cell trait is usually characterized by all of the following EXCEPT
   A. red cell concentration of S hemoglobin is about 40%
   B. splenic infarcts rarely occur except under extreme hypoxic conditions
   C. reticulocyte count is usually mildly elevated
   D. in some individuals, hyposthenuria and hematuria may result from sickling in the renal medullary capillaries
   E. the incidence in American blacks is one in 12

491. Which one of the following does NOT characterize heterozygous beta-thalassemia (minor or trait)?
   A. In most patients anemia and clinical symptoms are absent
   B. Life expectancy is shortened
   C. Varieties of this disorder are best distinguished by quantitation of A2 and F hemoglobins
   D. Peripheral blood examination reveals microcytosis, target cells, and variable degrees of hypochromia
   E. Severity depends on the degree of suppression of beta-globin synthesis

492. Beta-thalassemia major is associated with all of the following EXCEPT

A. defect in β-globin chain synthesis
B. the newborn infant is clinically and hematologically normal
C. the determination of A2 hemoglobin is important in diagnosis
D. onset of clinical symptoms and signs usually begins between six and 12 months of age
E. peripheral blood shows hypochromic and usually microcytic anemia

493. In hereditary spherocytosis, all of the following are characteristic EXCEPT

A. it is an autosomal dominant trait
B. there is loss of red cell membrane surface area without a reduction of cell volume, necessitating a spherical shape in order to accommodate its contents
C. spherocytes are more likely to rupture than normal cells when suspended in hypotonic solutions
D. the MCV is increased and the mean corpuscular hemoglobin concentration (MCHC) is decreased
E. clinical severity tends to be relatively consistent within families, although it varies widely from family to family

494. Vitamin E deficiency is associated with all of the following EXCEPT

A. greater prevalence in small premature infants
B. manifestation as normocytic normochromic anemia with an elevated reticulocyte count
C. acanthocytes are diagnostic
D. the only physical manifestations characteristic of this deficiency are edema of legs, labia, and eyelids in infants
E. it manifests itself as a mild hemolytic anemia

495. Characteristics of G6PD deficiency in patients include all of the following EXCEPT
   A. a sex-linked recessive pattern of inheritance
   B. persistence of low-grade anemia in patients
   C. the most common clinical manifestation is episodic acute hemolysis usually following infection or drug ingestion
   D. in blacks, G6PD activity is near normal in reticulocytes and young erythrocytes
   E. Heinz bodies are present only early in hemolytic episodes

496. Methemoglobinemia is associated with all of the following EXCEPT
   A. it is caused by oxidation of heme iron to the ferric state
   B. newborns are less susceptible because hemoglobin F is less rapidly oxidized to methemoglobin than is hemoglobin A
   C. M hemoglobinopathy, a form of methemoglobinemia, does not respond to methylene blue therapy
   D. a presumptive diagnosis can be made when fresh blood that is chocolate brown in color does not become red when aerated by mixing
   E. the discovery of clinical cyanosis is usually the first suggestion of this disorder

497. The Chediak–Higashi syndrome is characterized by all of the following EXCEPT
   A. neutropenia, probably the result of increased destruction of granulocytes within the bone marrow
   B. striking giant lysosomal granules present in neutrophils
   C. ability of neutrophils to phagocytose and kill bacteria normally
   D. albinism, photophobia, and nystagmus
   E. autosomal recessive mode of inheritance

498. Hodgkin disease is characterized by all of the following EXCEPT
   A. it is rare before five years of age
   B. the most common manifestation is painless, progressive enlargement of a lymph node
   C. involvement of axillary and cervical nodes are equal
   D. there is no characteristic abnormality of the blood
   E. Pel-Ebstein fever pattern

499. Non-Hodgkin lymphoma (formerly termed lymphosarcoma, reticulum cell sarcoma, or giant follicular lymphoma) differs from Hodgkin disease in all of the following EXCEPT
   A. in NHL, malignant cells appear more poorly undifferentiated
   B. NHL is three to four times more common
   C. dissemination occurs earlier and more often in NHL
   D. there is a greater female to male ratio in NHL
   E. therapy is less effective

500. Asplenism is associated with all of the following EXCEPT
   A. congenital absence occurs commonly with partial situs inversus
   B. fulminant infections occur most often in young children with infections due to *E. coli*
   C. it should be suspected in the presence of Howell–Jolly bodies on peripheral blood smear
   D. life-threatening infections are more commonly associated with sickle cell anemia than with postsplenectomy due to idiopathic thrombocytopenic purpura
   E. the risk of fulminant infection postsplenectomy never completely diminishes with age

501. The prothrombin time (PT) is a function of all of the following EXCEPT
   A. factor II
   B. factor V
   C. factor VII
   D. factor X
   E. factor IX

502. Partial thromboplastin time (PTT) is a function of all of the following EXCEPT
   A. factor VIII
   B. factor VII
   C. factor X
   D. factor XI
   E. factor IX

503. Vitamin K dependent factors include all of the following EXCEPT
   A. XI
   B. IX
   C. VII
   D. X
   E. II

504. Idiopathic thrombocytopenic purpura (ITP) is characterized by all of the following EXCEPT
   A. it is associated with antiplatelet antibody
   B. it frequently follows viral infection in children
   C. spontaneous remission is achieved by the great majority of cases
   D. prominent physical findings of splenomegaly are present
   E. bone marrow examination may reveal increased platelet production

505. Which of the following laboratory findings is NOT characteristic of ITP?
   A. Platelet count below 50,000/mm³
   B. Normal PT, PTT, normal thrombin time (TT)
   C. Normal WBC count
   D. Bone marrow reveals decreased number of megakaryocytes
   E. Clotting retraction is poor to absent

506. In hemolytic uremic syndrome all of the following are characteristic EXCEPT
A. bloody diarrhea
B. long-term sequelae are most often associated with the common neurologic manifestations
C. recurrent episodes are rare
D. hematuria
E. thrombocytopenia

507. Von Willebrand disease is characterized by all of the following EXCEPT
A. autosomal dominant inheritance
B. bleeding diathesis is usually manifested by hemarthrosis
C. reduction in plasma factor VIII
D. deficient platelet adhesion
E. menorrhagia may be a serious problem

508. Classic hemophilia is usually associated with all of the following EXCEPT
A. major joint hemarthroses are common
B. abnormal partial thromboplastin time
C. normal level of factor VIII antigen
D. abnormal clotting time
E. hematuria is a frequent manifestation

509. All of the following statements are true regarding factor XII deficiency (Hageman trait) EXCEPT
A. the bleeding problem is similar to factor XI deficiency
B. abnormal PTT
C. abnormal clotting time
D. abnormal prothrombin consumption test
E. patients are not subject to abnormal bleeding

510. Disseminated intravascular coagulation (DIC) may be associated with all of the following EXCEPT
A. the bleeding problem is similar to factor XI deficiency
B. abnormal PTT
C. abnormal clotting time
D. abnormal prothrombin consumption test
E. patients are not subject to abnormal bleeding

DIRECTIONS: Each set of lettered headings below is followed by a list of numbered words or phrases. For each numbered word or phrase select

A   if the item is associated with **A** only,
B   if the item is associated with **B** only,
C   if the item is associated with both **A** and **B**,
D   if the item is associated with neither **A** nor **B**.

A. Sickle cell disease
B. Thalassemia
C. Both
D. Neither

511. An abnormality of the erythrocyte membrane

512. Patients have high incidence of pneumococcal and Salmonella infections

513. Autosomal dominant mode of inheritance

514. Under normal circumstances heterozygotes have no symptoms

515. An abnormality of the structure of the beta-hemoglobin chain

A. Hemophilia A (classic hemophilia)
B. Von Willebrand disease
C. Both
D. Neither

516. Decreased factor VIII activity

517. X-linked recessive mode of inheritance

518. Associated with thrombocytopenia

519. Autosomal dominant mode of inheritance

520. Prolonged prothrombin time

DIRECTIONS: Each group of questions below consists of five lettered headings, followed by a list of numbered words, phrases or statements. For each numbered word, phrase or statement, select the **one** lettered heading that is most closely associated with it. Each lettered heading may be selected once, more than once, or not at all.

A. Enlarged spleen
B. Renal involvement
C. Repeated transfusions
D. Viral respiratory infection
E. Splenectomy indicated

521. Acute idiopathic thrombocytopenic purpura

522. Hereditary spherocytosis

523. Thalassemia major

524. Schönlein–Henoch syndrome

525. G6PD deficiency

Blood and Blood-Forming Tissues
Answers and Comments

469. C. This humoral substance is produced primarily in the kidney. (Ref. 1, p. 1035)

470. A. Hemoglobin A is alpha 2 beta 2; hemoglobin A2 is alpha 2 delta 2; hemoglobin Gower 2 is alpha 2 epsilon 2; and hemoglobin Gower 1 contains 4 epsilon chains. (Ref. 1, p. 1038)

471. D. The average volume is 75 to 77 ml/kg. (Ref. 1, p. 1037)

472. D. There is a shift to the right after owing to the decreased production of hemoglobin F, which has a lower affinity for 2,3 diphosphoglycerate (important in modulating the interaction between hemoglobin and oxygen). In the other three conditions mentioned, the shift results from an increase in RBC concentration of 2,3 DPG. (Ref. 1, p. 1039)

473. A. All the others are associated with a high MCV. (Ref. 1, p. 1041)

474. C. All others are usually associated with normal MCV and a low reticulocyte index. (Ref. 1, p. 1041)

475. D. An increase in serum unconjugated bilirubin is associated with extravascular hemolysis. (Ref. 1. p. 1042)

476. E. Absorption is decreased by formation of insoluble phosphates and oxalates, which is favored by the alkaline environment of the small intestine. (Ref. 1, p. 1045)

477. C. A low concentration has been found only in association with iron deficiency. (Ref. 1, p. 1046)

478. C. Hypersegmentation of neutrophils is easy to detect on peripheral blood smear. Even when deficiencies of both iron and folate coexist, hypersegmentation is usually present, whereas red cell indicies and serum folate levels become less reliable. (Ref. 1, p. 1049)

479. D. There is no clear inheritance pattern although endocrinopathies and immune deficiencies may be present in siblings. (Ref. 1, p. 1050)

480. A. Depression of serum vitamin B_{12} and the appearance of hypersegmented neutrophils are the earliest clinical manifestations. (Ref. 1, p. 1051)

481. C. The bone marrow stained for iron shows reduced or absent iron in erythroid precursors, despite the presence of RE iron. (Ref. 1, p. 1052)

482. A. Hepatomegaly is rare, adenopathy is absent, and splenomegaly is found in only 10% of cases. (Ref. 1, p. 1053)

483. D. Only about one in ten patients will develop acute leukemia. (Ref. 1, p. 1054)

484. C. Routine Rh testing generally fails to detect the D^u antigen because it is a weaker form of the D antigen and does not react with routine testing sera. The presence of D^u antigen means the mother is actually Rh-positive. (Ref. 1, p. 1057)

485. C. Islet cell hyperplasia and hyperinsulinism are present. It has been suggested that free hemoglobin in plasma binds to and inactivates insulin; the compensatory increase in insulin production causes islet cell hyperplasia. (Ref. 1, p. 1058)

486. C. Cephalothin usually results in a false positive Coombs test by the nonimmunologic adsorption of proteins on the surface of the red cell. This is not associated with hemolysis, and only in rare situations does it act as an hapten with resulting hemolysis. (Ref. 1, p. 1067)

487. B. Leukopenia and thrombocytopenia are commonly seen. (Ref. 1, p. 1068)

488. D. Hypertonicity of plasma increases intracellular concentration of hemoglobin S, and dehydration promotes sickling. (Ref. 1, p. 1068)

489. D. Salmonella osteomyelitis rarely progresses to sepsis. (Ref. 1, p. 1069)

490. C. The hemoglobin, hematocrit, and reticulocyte count are normal in sickle cell trait. (Ref. 1, p. 1072)

491. B. Life expectancy is normal. (Ref. 1, p. 1074)

492. C. The relative percentage of A2 hemoglobin may be reduced, normal, or elevated. Therefore, it is of little diagnostic value. (Ref. 1, p. 1075)

493. D. The MCV is at or below the lower limit of normal for age and the MCHC is greater than normal and often as high as 37%. (Ref. 1, p. 1078)

494. C. Red cell morphology is characterized by the presence of acanthocytes; however, they are also relatively common and reversible findings in infants with an adequate supply of vitamin E and, therefore, are of limited help in the diagnosis. (Ref. 1, p. 1081)

495. B. Between hemolytic episodes, anemia is absent, and RBC survival may be normal. (Ref. 1, p. 1083)

496. B. Newborns are more susceptible because hemoglobin F is more readily oxidized than hemoglobin A. (Ref. 1, p. 1087)

497. C. Neutrophils exhibit a delay in their ability to phagocytose and kill bacteria. (Ref. 1, p. 1093)

498. C. Sixty percent of the cases occur initially in the neck, with axillary and inguinal adenopathies less frequent. (Ref. 1, p. 1103)

499. D. As in Hodgkin disease, the male/female ratio is 3:1. (Ref. 1, p. 1105)

500. B. Pneumococci and *H. influenza* are responsible for most of the cases of sepsis in asplenia. (Ref. 1, p. 1108)

501. E. PT measures thrombin generation in the extrinsic pathway. Factor IX is part of the intrinsic clotting system. (Ref. 1, p. 1113)

502. B. PTT measures thrombin generation in the intrinsic pathway and is a function of all of the coagulation factors except factor VII. (Ref. 1, p. 1113)

503. A. Vitamin K dependent factors include factors II, VII, IX and X, which are low at birth and often fall to even lower levels during the first week unless vitamin K is given soon after birth. (Ref. 1, p. 1113)

504. D. Enlargement of spleen and lymph nodes is rare. (Ref. 1, p. 1115)

505. D. Bone marrow exam may reveal an increased number of megakaryocytes with a predominance of immature forms. (Ref. 1, p. 1116)

506. B. Long-term sequelae are restricted to chronic renal disease. (Ref. 1, p. 1117)

507. B. Nosebleeds and easy bruising are the most common manifestations; hemarthroses are rare. (Ref. 1, p. 1121)

508. D. Whole blood clotting time is markedly prolonged only in severe hemophilia; only 1% to 2% of normal factor VIII levels will produce a normal clotting time. (Ref. 1, p. 1119)

509. A. Patients are not subject to abnormal bleeding. The problem is usually found in screening tests for bleeding difficulties. (Ref. 1, p. 1121)

510. D. TT estimates the amount and function of fibrinogen and is particularly sensitive to the presence of fibrin degradation products, which are elevated in DIC. (Ref. 1, p. 1123)

511. **D.** Both sickle cell disease and thalassemia are abnormal-
512. **A.** ities of hemoglobin synthesis, and both are inherited as
513. **D.** autosomal recessive traits. Sickle cell patients have a
514. **A.** high incidence of pneumococcal and Salmonella infec-
515. **A.** tions, and the heterozygotes are asymptomatic. Sickle
cell has abnormalities of beta-chain synthesis only and they do not
involve the RBC membrane. (Ref. 1, pp. 1068–1076)

516. **C.** Hemophilia A has an X-linked mode of inheritance and
517. **A.** decreased factor VIII activity. Von Willebrand disease
518. **D.** is autosomal dominant and also has decreased factor
519. **B.** VIII activity. Neither is associated with thrombocyto-
520. **D.** penia or prolonged prothrombin times. (Ref. 1, pp.
1119–1121)

521. **D.**   ITP is associated with antecedent rubella or viral
522. **A,E.**   respiratory infection. Splenectomy is curative for
523. **A,C,E.** spherocytosis, but is reserved for only some chronic
524. **B.**   cases of ITP. Thalassemia major is treated by re-
525. **C.**   peated transfusions, and an enlarged spleen is a
characteristic clinical finding in this condition, sometimes necessitating removal because of mechanical discomfort or hypersplen-
ism. HS purpura has renal involvement in about 40% of cases.
G6PD deficiency may require transfusions if repeated episodes of
hemolysis are severe. The best approach is complete avoidance of
any drugs known to precipitate hemolytic crises. (Ref. 2, pp. 1218,
1222, 1227, 1248, 1338)

17 Kidney and Urinary Tract

DIRECTIONS: Each of the questions or incomplete statements below is followed by five suggested answers or completions. Select the **one** that is best in each case.

---

526. Urinary excretion of potassium is increased in all of the following EXCEPT
- **A.** persistent increased intake of potassium
- **B.** increased amounts of circulatory mineralocorticoid hormones
- **C.** metabolic acidosis
- **D.** administration of diuretics such as hydrochlorothiazide
- **E.** respiratory alkalosis

527. Orthostatic proteinuria is characterized by all of the following EXCEPT
- **A.** the usual age of detection is the second decade of life
- **B.** it is usually a subtle manifestation of chronic renal disease
- **C.** there is an increased amount of urinary protein when the patient is in upright position
- **D.** proteinuria is resolved when the patient is in a recumbent position
- **E.** total 24-hour urinary excretion of protein seldom exceeds 1000 mg

528. Which one of the following statements regarding hematuria is NOT true?
  - **A.** If casts are present the source of hematuria must be the kidney
  - **B.** Bright red urine which clots usually suggests renal or upper urinary tract source of bleeding
  - **C.** The additional finding of proteinuria usually suggests a renal source
  - **D.** The most common neoplasm associated with hematuria is Wilms tumor
  - **E.** It can be a cause of anemia

529. Which of the following findings is considered the essential common feature shared by all manifestations of the nephrotic syndrome?
  - **A.** Marked proteinuria
  - **B.** Hyperlipidemia
  - **C.** Hypertension
  - **D.** Hypoproteinemia
  - **E.** Edema

530. All of the following are consistent with the diagnosis of idiopathic nephrotic syndrome of childhood EXCEPT
  - **A.** onset is between two and eight years of age
  - **B.** pathologic renal changes are minimal by light microscopy
  - **C.** depression of C3
  - **D.** hypertension is unusual
  - **E.** hyperlipidemia

531. Acute poststreptococcal glomerulonephritis is characterized by all of the following EXCEPT
  - **A.** specific streptococcal antigens are found at the site of IgG and β 1c globulin deposits in the glomerulus
  - **B.** marked depression of C3 and terminal components of complement
  - **C.** prognosis is good due to the self-limited character of the nephritis
  - **D.** nephritis occurs in about 50% of children with anaphylactoid purpura
  - **E.** gross or microscopic hematuria

532. The nephritis of anaphylactoid purpura is manifested by all of the following EXCEPT
    A. severity of the nephritis correlates well with the amount of protein excreted
    B. serum β 1c globulin level is depressed
    C. prognosis is good, due to the self-limiting character of the nephritis
    D. nephritis occurs in about 50% of children with anaphylactoid purpura
    E. gross or microscopic hematuria

533. The pathophysiology of the hemolytic uremic syndrome is associated with all of the following EXCEPT
    A. immune mechanisms are considered important in the pathogenesis
    B. hemolytic anemia is Coombs negative
    C. thrombocytopenia probably results from platelet aggregation within damaged vessels
    D. renal microangiopathy affecting small arterioles and glomerular capillaries is the most consistent pathologic change
    E. uncertain pathogenesis

534. Renal tubular acidosis (RTA) may be accurately described by and associated with all of the following EXCEPT
    A. a clinical syndrome of sustained hyperchloremic metabolic acidosis in the absence of significant reduction in glomerular filtration rate
    B. distal and proximal RTA occur either as primary abnormalities in urine acidification or as secondary disorders to systemic disease or intoxication
    C. distal RTA, compared to proximal RTA, is more commonly secondary to a systemic disorder or toxin
    D. nephrocalcinosis is seen in distal RTA
    E. failure to thrive

535. Nephrogenic diabetes insipidus is associated with all of the following EXCEPT
    A. unresponsiveness of proximal tubule to vasopressin
    B. decreased production of cyclic 3,5-AMP which mediates the permeability of distal tubule to the passive diffusion of luminal water into medullary interstitium
    C. normal transport of tubular sodium and chloride
    D. no consistent renal pathological changes are demonstrated
    E. hypernatremia

536. Renal glycosuria may be characterized by all of the following EXCEPT
    A. hereditary defect in tubular glucose transport
    B. glucose tolerance curve is either normal or flat
    C. urinary loss of glucose has little effect on blood glucose concentration
    D. all urine specimens contain glucose regardless of normal blood glucose concentrations
    E. inherited usually as sex linked

537. Which one of the following is NOT associated with Alport syndrome?
    A. Most common of the heritable renal diseases
    B. High frequency of sensorineural deafness
    C. Cataracts
    D. Wide geographic distributions are found in patients of different racial and ethnic backgrounds
    E. Onset during the second decade

538. Childhood polycystic kidney disease is characterized by all of the following EXCEPT
    A. liver involvement is common and is associated with dilatation of portal bile ducts
    B. renal disease presenting at adolescence or later is relatively milder than that in infants
    C. it is an autosomal recessive disorder
    D. associated lower urinary system abnormalities are common
    E. hematuria may be present

539. Acute pyelonephritis in children is associated with all of the following EXCEPT

    A. impaired migration of polymorphonuclear leukocytes and phagocytosis because of medullary hypertonicity

    B. it is often secondary to reflux from lower urinary tract

    C. impaired ability to concentrate

    D. it is rarely associated with meatal stenosis

    E. abdominal pain

540. Renal vein thrombosis in infants is characterized by all of the following EXCEPT

    A. it is probably related to venous stasis secondary to shock, septicemia, or dehydration

    B. edema and hypertension

    C. thrombocytopenia

    D. disseminated intravascular coagulopathy

    E. an enlarged kidney that does not visualize on intravenous urography

---

DIRECTIONS: Each group of questions below consists of five lettered headings followed by a list of numbered words, phrases, or statements. For each numbered word, phrase, or statement, select the **one** lettered heading that is most closely associated with it. Each lettered heading may be selected once, more than once, or not at all.

    A. Goodpasture syndrome

    B. Hemolytic-uremic syndrome

    C. Systemic lupus erythematosus

    D. Acute poststreptococcal glomerulonephritis

    E. Polyarteritis nodosa

541. Majority of patients have no permanent impairment of renal function

542. Associated with nephritis and pulmonary hemorrhage

543. The female/male ratio for this type of nephritis is 4:1

544. Thought to be a hypersensitivity reaction involving medium-sized vessels in its chronic form

545. Usually preceded by a gastroenteritis prodrome

546. Steroids and cytotoxic immunosuppressant drugs are now recommended as therapy

    A. Hydrocele
    B. Posterior urethral valves
    C. Horseshoe kidney
    D. Prune belly syndrome
    E. Vesicourethral reflux

547. Absence of abdominal wall musculature, bilateral undescended testes, and urinary tract anomalies

548. Found in high frequency in patients with Turner syndrome

549. Spontaneous cure is likely and usually occurs in the first year of life

550. Provides a ready pathway for ascending urinary tract infections

551. A congenital abnormality of the verumontanum

552. Transillumination can be diagnostic

    A. Glycosuria
    B. Proteinuria
    C. Alkaline urine pH
    D. Hematuria
    E. Low specific gravity

553. Poststreptococcal glomerulonephritis

554. Distal renal tubular acidosis

555. Minimum change nephrotic syndrome

556. Fanconi syndrome

557. Nephrogenic diabetes insipidus

Kidney and Urinary Tract
Answers and Comments

526. C. Potassium excretion is reduced during respiratory and metabolic acidosis. During alkalosis hydrogen is exchanged for potassium; therefore, the amount of potassium available for secretion increases, and the excretion is enhanced. (Ref. 2, p. 1312)

527. B. May be normal variant and most children are healthy and have no underlying renal pathology. (Ref. 2, p. 1310)

528. B. Bright red urine, with or without clots, suggests an extrarenal source of bleeding. (Ref. 2, p. 1310)

529. A. Proteinuria usually to the extent of 2 $g/m^2/24$ hrs or more. (Ref. 2, p. 1308)

530. C. Serum level of C3 is usually normal. Additionally, immunopathologic studies reveal an absence of deposits of immune globulins or complement components. (Ref. 2, p. 1322)

531. A. Specific streptococcal antigens are not found at the site of IgG and β lc deposition. (Ref. 2, p. 1331)

532. B. Serum β lc level is normal. Glomerular deposits of IgG and β lc have been seen but do not have characteristic location or appearance seen in other forms of immune complex injury. (Ref. 2, p. 1338)

533. A. Immune mechanisms are not considered operative, since there is no deposition of complement components or immunoglobulins at the site of the arteriolar or glomerular lesions. (Ref. 2, p. 1340)

534. C. Proximal RTA also occurs as a primary isolated defect, but is more commonly secondary to a systemic disorder or toxin. It is usually associated with other features of impaired tubular transport. (Ref. 2, p. 1344)

535. A. Primary defect is believed to be an enzymatic or biochemical abnormality in distal tubular function. (Ref. 2, p. 1347)

536. E. In some families the condition is inherited as an autosomal dominant, in others an autosomal recessive mode is probable. (Ref. 2, p. 1349)

537. E. The mean age of onset is six years, but it has been noted as early as five months. (Ref. 2, p. 1350)

538. D. The renal pelvicies, ureters, bladder, and urethra are normal. (Ref. 2, p. 1356)

539. C. Decreasing concentrating ability is usually associated with chronic pyelonephritis and is most likely a result of damage to the renal medulla, progressive interstitial scarring, and nephron destruction. (Ref. 2, p. 1367)

540. B. Edema and hypertension are usually absent. (Ref. 2, p. 1378)

541. D. The ratio of females to males with SLE is 4:1. It is now
542. A. recommended that SLE patients with renal involvement
543. C. be treated with steroids, and if no response is observed,
544. E. cytotoxic immunosuppressants are used. Goodpasture
545. B. syndrome is associated with nephritis and pulmonary
546. C. hemorrhage. In the hemolytic uremic syndrome there is usually a prodrome of gastroenteritis. The pathology of chronic polyarteritis nodosa involves a hypersensitivity reaction of the medium-sized vessel. The majority of patients with acute poststreptococcal glomerulonephritis recover without permanent renal damage, unlike the other listed conditions. (Ref. 1, pp. 1184–1188)

547. D. Hydroceles can be diagnosed by physical examination
548. C. and transillumination and carry a high spontaneous cure
549. A. rate during the first year of life. The prune belly triad
550. E. consists of absence of abdominal muscles, undescended
551. B. testes, and various renal abnormalities. Vesicoureteral
552. A. reflux provides a ready pathway for bacteria in ascending urinary tract infection. Posterior urethral valves are a congenital

malformation of the verumontanum. Horseshoe kidneys are found with high frequency with Turner syndrome. (Ref. 1, pp. 1220–1223)

553. **B,D.**   Acute glomerulonephritis may be complicated by
554. **C,E.**   hypertensive encephalopathy, heart failure, or
555. **B.**   acute renal failure. Distal RTA consists of sys-
556. **A,B,C,E.** temic acidosis and failure to thrive due to an in-
557. **E.**   ability to reabsorb bicarbonate, with secondary
damage from nephrocalcinosis and hypokalemia resulting in impaired concentrating ability. Minimum change nephrotic syndrome consists of proteinuria, hypoproteinemia, edema and hyperlipidemia. Hematuria is present in less than 10% of cases. The disease is usually responsive to steroids. Fanconi syndrome produces rickets and growth retardation in addition to a multitude of problems secondary to proximal RTA, and excessive excretion of sodium and potassium. (Ref. 2, pp. 1324, 1330, 1345, 1347)

18 Bones and Joints

558. Components of congenital clubfoot include all of the following EXCEPT
    A. metatarsus adductus
    B. calcaneovalgus
    C. plantar flexion
    D. equinovarus deformity of the ankle
    E. relative rigidity of position

559. The most common organism associated with osteomyelitis in children is
    A. *S. aureus*
    B. group A beta-hemolytic streptococcus
    C. Salmonella
    D. *H. influenzae*
    E. *Streptococcus viridans*

560. All of the following are characteristic of cleidocranial dysplasia EXCEPT
A. poorly formed dentition
B. widely spaced eyes
C. failure of development of the clavicle
D. soft calvarium
E. mental retardation

561. Marfan syndrome and homocystinuria share all of the following clinical features EXCEPT
A. mental retardation
B. ectopia lentis
C. skeletal deformities
D. excessive length of tubular bones
E. genetic transmission to offspring

562. Coxa plana (Legg–Calve–Perthes disease) is characterized by all of the following EXCEPT
A. limitation of abduction and of external rotation of the hip
B. it rarely develops before three years of age
C. hip pain is frequently referred to the medial side of the ipsilateral knee
D. it is more frequent in boys than girls
E. bilateral hip involvement occurs in the majority of cases

563. Infantile cortical hyperostosis is characterized by all of the following EXCEPT
A. high erythrocyte sedimentation rate
B. increased alkaline phosphatase
C. lymphadenopathy
D. external thickening of bony cortex
E. negative bacterial, viral, and serologic studies

564. Which of the following organisms is associated most often in acute pyarthrosis in children under two years?
A. *S. aureus*
B. Beta-hemolytic streptococci
C. Pneumococci
D. *H. influenzae*
E. *S. viridans*

DIRECTIONS: Each group of questions below consists of five lettered headings followed by a list of numbered words, phrases, or statements. For each numbered word, phrase, or statement, select the **one** lettered heading that is most closely associated with it. Each lettered heading may be selected once, more than once, or not at all.

A. Osgood-Schlatter disease
B. Subluxation of the head of the radius
C. Legg-Calve-Perthes disease
D. Slipped femoral epiphysis
E. Congenital subluxation of the hip

565. Aseptic necrosis of the capital femoral epiphysis

566. Benign condition completely resolved after simple reduction

567. Believed to be caused by chronic trauma to the anterior tibial tubercle

568. Associated with Ortolani's click

569. Occurs typically in the "overlarge" adolescent with the insidious onset of knee pain

570. Disease of unknown cause occurring most frequently in males between the ages of four and 10 years

A. Apert syndrome
B. Neurofibromatosis
C. Klippel–Feil syndrome
D. Kohler disease
E. Poland syndrome

571. Osteochondritis of the tarsonavicular bone

572. Syndactyly and premature closure of the coronal sutures

573. Pseudarthrosis of the tibia

574. Absence of the second to fourth ribs and pectoralis muscle

575. Failure of segmentation of the cervical spine

Bones and Joints
Answers and Comments

558. B. Calcaneovalgus refers to dorsiflexion with lateral deviation; the opposite is the case in clubfoot. (Ref. 1, p. 1823)

559. A. *S. aureus* accounts for 70% to 90% of cases in otherwise normal children. (Ref. 1, p. 1830)

560. E. Intelligence is normal. Despite the softness of the calvarium, it rarely results in brain damage. Convulsive disorders and development of neurologic abnormalities occasionally occur. (Ref. 1, p. 365)

561. A. Universal mental retardation and urinary excretion of homocystine are features of homocystinuria. In addition the latter is transmitted as an autosomal recessive trait as opposed to autosomal dominant in Marfan syndrome. (Ref. 1, p. 372)

562. E. Bilateral involvement occurs in only 10% of cases. (Ref. 1, p. 1834)

563. C. There is no lymphadenopathy in any phase of the disease. (Ref. 1, p. 370)

564. D. Staphylococci are most often found in children over two years of age. (Ref. 1, p. 535)

565. C. Legg-Calve-Perthes disease is of unknown etiology and
566. B. most commonly affects males between four and ten years
567. A. of age. The lesion found is aseptic necrosis of the hip.
568. E. Slipped capital femoral epiphysis occurs with insidious
569. D. onset of knee pain in the "overlarge" adolescent. Sub-
570. C. luxation of the head of the radius is a benign condition.
Congenital subluxation of the hip is suggested by a click felt while performing the Ortolani maneuver. Osgood-Schlatter disease is believed to be caused by chronic trauma to the tibial tubercle. (Ref. 2, pp. 1614–1621)

571. D. Kohler disease is an osteochondritis of the tarso navi-
572. A. cular bone. Premature closure of the coronal with syn-
573. B. dactyly is known as Apert syndrome. It is believed to
574. E. be transmitted on an autosomal dominant basis, and may
575. C. involve syndactyly of the feet as well. Neurofibromatosis
is associated with pseudo-arthrosis of the tibia. Poland syndrome
involves rib dysplasia and absence of one or both pectoralis muscles
on the affected side. Klippel-Feil syndrome requires no treatment,
and may be associated with Sprengel deformity. (Ref. 3, pp. 397–
403)

19 Eye

DIRECTIONS: Each of the questions or incomplete statements below is followed by five suggested answers or completions. Select the **one** that is best in each case.

576. The normal child has a visual acuity approximating that of the adult (20/20) at age
    A. seven to eight weeks
    B. three to four months
    C. 18 to 24 months
    D. two to three years
    E. four to five years

577. All of the following are correct statements regarding color vision EXCEPT
    A. color vision deficits may lead to learning disturbances in school
    B. color blindness is usually partial
    C. color blindness is usually of the red-green deficiency type
    D. color blindness is no longer recognized as a sex-linked disorder
    E. there is no suitable treatment for color blindness

225

578. Leukokoria is associated with
   A. retinoblastoma
   B. interstitial keratitis
   C. ocular albinism
   D. conjunctivitis
   E. blepharitis

579. The most common anomaly of the eyelids is
   A. entropion
   B. congenital ptosis
   C. ectropion
   D. palpebral coloboma
   E. blepharophimosis

580. A child is seen with a very peculiar form of eyelid ptosis. When the mouth is opened or when the jaw is moved to the side opposite the ptosis, there is elevation of the ptotic lid. This is called
   A. Marcus Gunn phenomenon
   B. trichiasis
   C. Waardenburg syndrome
   D. epicanthal phenomenon
   E. Horner syndrome

581. A child presents with scaling and inflammation of the mucocutaneous borders of the angles of the lids. Microscopic examination of the scrapings reveals large gram-negative diplobacilli with no leukocytes. The most likely diagnosis is infection with
   A. *S. aureus*
   B. *Moraxella lacunata*
   C. *Pediculus pubis*
   D. *P. capitis*
   E. *N. gonorrhea*

582. All of the following are true statements about trachoma
    EXCEPT
    A. it is the most common cause of impaired vision
    B. in some localities it is endemic
    C. it is caused by herpes simplex
    D. the acute phase is followed by a chronic low-grade
        inflammation
    E. corticosteroids are contraindicated

583. Dislocation of the lens has been associated with all of the
    following EXCEPT
    A. Marchesani syndrome
    B. arachnodactyly
    C. homocystinuria
    D. maternal rubella
    E. trauma

584. The earliest and most common finding associated with in-
    fantile congenital glaucoma is
    A. tearing
    B. photophobia
    C. strabismus
    D. cupping of the optic disc
    E. megalocornea

DIRECTIONS: Each set of lettered headings below is followed by
a list of numbered words or phrases. For each numbered word or
phrase select
    A   if the item is associated with A only,
    B   if the item is associated with B only,
    C   if the item is associated with both A and B,
    D   if the item is associated with neither A nor B.

    A. Gonococcal ophthalmia neonatorum
    B. Inclusion blenorrhea
    C. Both
    D. Neither

585. Prevented by silver nitrate prophylaxis

586. Associated with redness and swelling of the lids and profuse exudate

587. Systemic antibiotics are indicated

588. High morbidity even with adequate therapy

589. Causative organism is acquired from the genital tract

    A. Cataract
    B. Uveitis
    C. Both
    D. Neither

590. May be caused by *Toxocara canis*

591. Seen in patients with galactosemia

592. After trauma to one eye, it may appear in the previously unaffected eye

593. Frequently seen in congenital rubella infection

594. Can be a cause of blindness

DIRECTIONS: Each group of questions below consists of lettered headings, followed by a list of numbered words, phrases or statements. For each numbered word, phrase or statement, select the **one** lettered heading that is most closely associated with it. Each lettered heading may be selected once, more than once, or not at all.

    A. Cherry red spot in macula
    B. Amblyopia ex anopsia
    C. Aniridia
    D. Nyctalopia
    E. Miosis
    F. Photophobia

595. Strabismus

596. Horner syndrome

597. Tay-Sachs disease

598. Wilms tumor

599. Vitamin A deficiency

Eye
Answers and Comments

576. E. The child at age four to five years has a visual acuity level like that of the adult (20/20). At birth the visual acuity is approximately 20/400. By age three to four years the child can be tested with the Snellen E chart. (Ref. 1, p. 1779)

577. D. Color vision deficiency is a sex-linked recessive disorder. It occurs in 7.5% of white males, 4% of black males, and only 0.6% of all girls. (Ref. 1, p. 1779)

578. A. Leukokoria (white pupillary reflex) is caused by several intraocular diseases but is most often seen with cataract, retinoblastoma, nematode endophthalmitis, and retrolental fibroplasia. (Ref. 1, p. 1800)

579. B. Drooping of the upper lid is usually unilateral but not uncommonly it is bilateral, and is secondary to defective development, or absence, of the muscle of the eyelid (the levator muscle). The deficit may be inherited as an autosomal dominant trait. (Ref. 1, p. 1783)

580. A. The Marcus Gunn phenomenon results from an anomalous connection between the external pterygoid muscle and the levator muscle. (Ref. 1, p. 1783)

581. B. The clinical description and microscopic findings are most compatible with angular blepharitis caused by *Moraxella lacunata* (formerly *H. duplex*). A type of squamous blepharitis, the organism described is also called the diplobacillus of Morax-Axenfeld. (Ref. 1, p. 1785)

582. C. The offending organism in trachoma is a virus that belongs to the psittacosis lymphogranuloma venerum group: *chlamydia*. Corticosteroids reactivate this organism and are contraindicated. (Ref. 1, p. 1788)

583. D. Maternal rubella is not usually associated with dislocation of the lens; it is associated with congenital cataract. (Ref. 2, p. 1759)

584. A. Tearing is the most common sign. The increased intra-ocular pressure may be present at birth or become apparent in the first three years of life. The tearing must be differentiated from congenital obstruction of the nasolacrimal duct. (Ref. 2, p. 1767)

585. A. Both gonococcal ophthalmia and inclusion blenorrhea
586. C. are associated with acute redness and swelling of the lids
587. C. and the production of exudate and both are acquired
588. D. from the genital tract. Neither is associated with great
589. C. morbidity after adequate therapy. In both, systemic an-tibiotics are indicated, but silver nitrate prophylaxis is effective in protecting against gonorrhea only. (Ref. 1, p. 1786)

590. B. Both cataracts and uveitis can be a cause of blindness.
591. A. Cataracts are frequently seen in patients with galacto-
592. B. semia and in congenital rubella, but uveitis is not. Uvei-
593. A. tis may be caused by Toxocara infection and may be
594. C. seen in the unaffected eye after trauma to the other eye. Cataracts are not seen in these circumstances. (Ref. 1, pp. 1796–1799)

595. B. Strabismus if not corrected early, may lead to loss of
596. E. vision in the deviating eye, in order to avoid diplopia.
597. A. Horner syndrome consists of homolateral ptosis, miosis,
598. C. and decreased facial sweating. It is caused by birth
599. D. trauma, or secondary to mass lesion in the brain stem, upper spinal cord, neck, middle fossa, or orbit. Tay-Sachs disease is a sphingolipidosis, which has a macular red spot, in addition to optic atrophy and progressive loss of vision. Photophobia, nystagmus, and defective vision are characteristics of aniridia. When sporadic, it is associated with an increased incidence of Wilms tumor. Nyctalopia or night blindness is a characteristic of vitamin A deficiency. (Ref. 2, pp. 1738, 1742, 1749–1751)

20 Ear, Nose, and Throat

DIRECTIONS: Each of the questions or incomplete statements below is followed by five suggested answers or completions. Select the **one** that is best in each case.

---

600. Kartagener syndrome is characterized by all of the following EXCEPT
    A. situs inversus
    B. bronchiectasis
    C. chronic sinusitis
    D. choanal atresia
    E. aplasia of the frontal sinuses

601. The most common malignant tumor observed in the nose and paranasal sinuses of children is
    A. rhabdomyosarcoma
    B. olfactory epithelioma
    C. lymphoma
    D. renal metastatic tumor
    E. angiofibromas

602. Waardenburg syndrome is associated with all of the following EXCEPT
    A. congenital deafness
    B. heterochromia of the iris
    C. narrow nasal bridge
    D. white forlock
    E. autosomal dominant inheritance

603. Pendred syndrome is associated with all of the following EXCEPT
  A. congenital deafness
  B. autosomal recessive inheritance
  C. goiter
  D. retinitis pigmentosa
  E. thyroid abnormality due to inability to change inorganic to organic iodide

604. Which one of the following does NOT characterize Treacher Collins syndrome?
  A. Autosomal dominant with variable penetrance
  B. Antimongoloid slanting of the eyes
  C. Neurosensory hearing loss
  D. Hypoplasia of facial bone
  E. Coloboma

605. Which one of the following does NOT characterize Alport syndrome?
  A. Autosomal dominant inheritance with variable penetrance
  B. Progressive high-tone hearing loss
  C. Glomerulonephritis
  D. Renal tubular acidosis
  E. Variable age on onset and rate of progression

606. Ramsey Hunt syndrome is associated with all of the following EXCEPT
  A. herpes zoster
  B. neurosensory deafness
  C. facial paralysis
  D. bullous myringitis
  E. involvement of the external auditory canal

DIRECTIONS: Each set of lettered headings below is followed by a list of numbered words or phrases. For each numbered word or phrase select

A   if the item is associated with **A** only,
B   if the item is associated with **B** only,
C   if the item is associated with both **A** and **B**,
D   if the item is associated with neither **A** nor **B**.

A. Peritonsillar abscess
B. Retropharyngeal abscess
C. Both
D. Neither

607. Incision and drainage is indicated

608. Predominant causative organism is group A beta-hemolytic strep

609. Steroids are important to reduce swelling and promote healing

610. A valid indication for tonsillectomy

611. Classically presents with fever, dysphagia, and trismus

Ear, Nose, and Throat
Answers and Comments

600. D. Choanal atresia is the most common congenital malformation of the nose, but is not part of Kartagener syndrome. (Ref. 1, p. 1431)

601. A. Malignant tumors are rare in the nose and parasinuses in children but, when present, the most common is the rhabdomyosarcoma. (Ref. 1, p. 902)

602. C. There is lateral displacement of the inner canthi of the eyes and a prominent broad nasal root. (Ref. 1, p. 891)

603. D. Retinitis pigmentosa associated with deafness is known as Usher syndrome. (Ref. 1, pp. 891, 1525)

604. C. Hearing loss is usually conductive because of the malformation of the external auditory canal and middle ear. (Ref. 1, p. 890)

605. D. Renal tubular acidosis with neurosensory hearing loss may be seen in autosomal recessive disease. (Ref. 1, p. 891)

606. D. The tympanic membrane is usually not involved in this viral infection. (Ref. 1, p. 895)

607. C. Incision and drainage is indicated in both of these dis-
608. C. eases, which are usually caused by group A beta-he-
609. D. molytic strep. Steroids have no place in their therapy.
610. A. One of the valid indications for tonsillectomy is a history
611. A. of peritonsillar abscess. Retropharyngeal abscess presents with hyperextension of the neck and noisy respirations in the patient, as opposed to the signs given for peritonsillar abscess. (Ref. 3, p. 98 and Ref. 2, p. 1017)

21 Skin

DIRECTIONS: Each of the questions or incomplete statements below is followed by five suggested answers or completions. Select the **one** that is best in each case.

---

612. The characteristics of dermatitis herpetiformis include all of the following EXCEPT
    A. occurrence in generally healthy children
    B. blood eosinophilia is common
    C. it is caused by herpes virus
    D. the grouped, symmetrical vesicles, or bullae, frequently exacerbate and then go into remission spontaneously
    E. urticarial lesions may predominate in mild cases

613. Toxic epidermal necrolysis (scalded skin syndrome, Lyell disease) is associated with all of the following EXCEPT
    A. it is most common in infants and young children
    B. group A beta-hemolytic streptococcus is the etiologic agent
    C. the entire skin, including palms and soles, may be involved as well as mucous membranes
    D. in children the clinical course is characterized by spontaneous improvement
    E. Nikolsky sign is positive

614. Erythema multiforme is characterized by all of the following EXCEPT
   A. relatively asymptomatic skin lesions
   B. with involvement of conjunctivitis and mucous membranes, the disease is sometimes called the Stevens-Johnson syndrome
   C. lesions, include macules, purpuric spots, urticaria, vesicles, and bullae
   D. the cause is unknown in most cases
   E. polymorphonuclear leukocytes usually predominant in the vesicular fluid

615. Cellulitis occurring about the face in young children (six to 24 months) and associated with fever and a purple skin discoloration is most often caused by
   A. group A beta-hemolytic streptococci
   B. *H. influenzae*
   C. *S. pneumococci*
   D. *S. aureus*
   E. *Pseudomonas*

616. Herpes zoster is associated with all of the following EXCEPT
   A. demonstration of intracytoplasmic inclusions by biopsy of lesions
   B. antibody may be found in both "slow" and "fast" IgG components
   C. persistent or severe pain during active disease is unusual in children, and postherpetic neuralgia is rare in childhood
   D. lesions characterized by grouped vesicles are located in the distribution of the infected spinal or cranial sensory nerves
   E. Guillain–Barré syndrome

617. Molluscum contagiosum is characterized by all of the following EXCEPT
   A. its only natural host is man
   B. unknown etiology
   C. lesions are discrete, nearly gray, umbilicated papules
   D. autoinoculation is common
   E. may appear at any age

618. Tinea capitis is associated with all of the following EXCEPT
   A. it is most often due to infection with microsporum species
   B. the lesions frequently fluoresce with Wood's lamp examination
   C. it is occasionally associated with kerion
   D. may be transmitted from animals to man
   E. easily treated with local fungistatic preparations

619. Incontinentia pigmenti is characterized by all of the following EXCEPT
   A. it occurs almost exclusively in males
   B. irregular whorled patterns of pigmentation
   C. dental abnormalities
   D. disorders of the central nervous system
   E. first signs of the disease are linear or grouped vesicles

620. Pityriasis rosea is characterized by all of the following EXCEPT
   A. it is a papulosquamous disease primarily of the trunk
   B. herald patch
   C. pruritus is most common symptom
   D. prodrome of cough, fever, and conjunctivitis
   E. color, distribution, and morphology of the lesions are usually sufficient to establish a diagnosis

DIRECTIONS: For each of the questions or imcomplete statements below, **one or more** of the answers or completions given is correct. Select

A   if only, **1, 2,** and **3** are correct,
B   if only **1** and **3** are correct,
C   if only **2** and **4** are correct,
D   if only **4** is correct,
E   if all are correct.

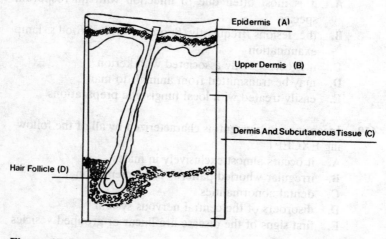

Epidermis (A)

Upper Dermis (B)

Dermis And Subcutaneous Tissue (C)

Hair Follicle (D)

Figure 17 Pyoderma may affect each of the illustrated levels (A-D) of the skin.

621.   In the approach to the patient with pyoderma (Fig. 17)
     1.   the infection should be considered to be mixed with both staph and strep present
     2.   septicemia should be considered a common problem
     3.   systemic antibiotics are considered to be superior to local therapy
     4.   family screening for carriers is not necessary

622.   Erythema multiforme has been associated with
     1.   streptococcal infections
     2.   drug sensitization
     3.   connective tissue diseases
     4.   tuberculosis

623. Vascular nevi that require no treatment and usually resolve spontaneously include
1. cavernous hemangioma
2. nevus araneus
3. nevus flammeus
4. strawberry hamangioma

624. Patients with eczema have been shown to have
1. family history of atopy
2. hyperactive T cells
3. abnormal response to intracutaneous methacholine
4. abnormal macrophage inhibitory factor (MIF) response

625. Conditions associated with hypopigmentation include
1. Waardenburg syndrome
2. Mucha-Habermann disease
3. Chédiak-Higashi syndrome
4. ephelides

DIRECTIONS: Each group of questions below consists of five lettered headings, followed by a list of numbered words, phrases or statements. For each numbered word, phrase or statement, select the **one** lettered heading that is most closely associated with it. Each lettered heading may be selected once, more than once, or not at all.

A. Erythrasma
B. Nevus simplex
C. Acrodermatitis enteropathica
D. Epidermal nevus
E. Dermatitis herpetiformis

626. Associated with seizures

627. Associated with gluten sensitive enteropathy

628. Associated with Corynebacterium minutissimum

629. Transient benign lesion

630. Associated with chronic diarrhea and perioral and perineal vesicobullous lesions

Skin
Answers and Comments

612. C. The etiology is unknown, although it is thought not to be an infectious process. (Ref. 1, p. 832)

613. B. Lyell disease is most often associated with a toxin from the coagulase positive phage group 2 staphylococci. (Ref. 1, p. 832)

614. E. Eosinophils may be present, but lymphocytes usually predominate. (Ref. 1, p. 831)

615. B. Cellulitis caused by staphylococci and streptococcal disease is usually associated with pyoderma (papulovesicular lesions). Pneumococcal infections are rarely associated with cellulitis. Pseudomonal infections associated with septicemia may be seen in ulcerative lesions. (Ref. 1, p. 835)

616. A. Inclusion bodies are intranuclear in zoster but are intracytoplasmic in smallpox. (Ref. 1, p. 613)

617. B. Molluscum is classified as a poxvirus. (Ref. 1, p. 833)

618. E. Infection of the hair and hair shafts usually requires systemic administration of griseofulvin. (Ref. 1, p. 838)

619. A. Occurs almost exclusively in infant females. (Ref. 1, p. 847)

620. D. Prodrome is rare but may be infrequently associated with low-grade fever and sore throat. (Ref. 1, p. 851)

621. B. Pyoderma is usually a mixed infection of both staph and strep. Systemic antibiotics are far superior to local therapy. Family contacts should be screened to detect carriers. Sepsis is an uncommon complication of pyoderma. (Ref. 1, p. 834)

622. E. All of the conditions listed have been associated with erythema multiforme as have mycoplasma, herpes simplex, and deep mycoses. (Ref. 1, p. 831)

623. C. Cavernous hemangioma and nevus flammeus (port wine stain) do not resolve spontaneously. (Ref. 1, p. 853)

624. B. Patients with eczema have been shown to have a high incidence of family history of atopy and an abnormal methacholine test as evidenced by delayed blanching. (Ref. 1, p. 849)

625. B. Waardenburg and Chédiak-Higashi syndromes are associated with patterned leukoderma and albinism, respectively. Mucha-Habermann disease and ephelides (freckles) are not associated with hypopigmentation. (Ref. 1, p. 845)

626. D. Epidermal nevi may be isolated, or associated with other
627. E. abnormalities, such as hemangiomas, ocular defects,
628. A. Wilms tumor, as well as neurologic defects. Dermatitis
629. B. herpetiformis is characterized by symmetrical, grouped
630. C. vesicular, puritic lesions of unknown etiology. Erythrasma is a chronic superficial infection, most common in adolescents, which responds well to erythromycin. Nevus simplex, also known as a salmon patch, are very common lesions found in newborns, especially on the eyelids, upper lip, and nuchal area. Acrodermatitis enteropathica responds to zinc therapy. (Ref. 2, pp. 1666, 1675, 1683, 1684, 1714)

22 Teeth

DIRECTIONS: Each of the questions or incomplete statements below is followed by five suggested answers or completions. Select the **one** that is best in each case.

---

631. In regard to the eruption of teeth, which of the following situations is ABNORMAL?
     A. First tooth at four months
     B. First tooth at six months
     C. First tooth at eight months
     D. Permanent central incisor at seven months
     E. First tooth at 16 months

632. All of the following might be possible etiologies for discoloration of the teeth of a 15-month-old infant EXCEPT
     A. iron medication
     B. dental decay
     C. tetracycline given to mother during pregnancy
     D. breastfeeding
     E. improper fluoride administration

633. Nighttime bottle caries can be prevented by
     A. toothbrushing in the morning
     B. the substitution of juice for milk
     C. only using milk in the bottle
     D. using only sugar water at naptime
     E. not giving a bottle at naptime or bedtime

Table 11 Recommended Dosage Levels of Supplemental Fluoride

Age (yr)	Drinking Water Fluoride Concentration, ppm		
	0.0–0.3 (mg/day)	0.3–0.7 (mg/day)	0.7+ (mg/day)
0–2	0.25	0.0	0.0
2–3	0.50	0.25	0.0
3–13	1.00	0.50	0.0

634. Fluoridation of the water supply (Table 11) has been associated with

   A. a reduction in decay of more than 60%

   B. overall support of the practice by the dental and medical professions

   C. increased incidence of early dental eruption

   D. increased incidence of delayed dental eruption

   E. no appreciable reduction in decay

Teeth
Answers and Comments

631. E. Infrequently the first tooth will not erupt until 12 months of age. Eruption occurring later than this would require investigation. (Ref. 1, p. 874)

632. D. Other causes of dental discoloration include trauma, and tetracycline administration before the age of eight years. (Ref. 2, p. 1022)

633. E. Any sugar-containing fluid nursed by the infant at nap-time or nighttime is a potential caries producer. The upper teeth usually show signs of disease before the lower teeth. The syndrome has *not* been reported in infants who breastfeed frequently at night. (Ref. 1, p. 881)

634. A. While not all professional health groups are convinced of the safety and efficacy of fluoridation, studies demonstrate significant reduction in dental decay. (Ref. 1, p. 880)

23 Unclassified Disorders

DIRECTIONS: Each of the questions or incomplete statements below is followed by five suggested answers or completions. Select the **one** that is best in each case.

---

635. Which of the following factors is NOT associated with increased risk of sudden infant death syndrome?
    A. Lower socioeconomic status
    B. Illegitimate birth
    C. Young mother with high parity
    D. Infant age of two to four months
    E. Spotting during the first trimester

636. Patients with familial Mediterranean fever display all of the following EXCEPT
    A. a positive rectal biopsy for amyloid
    B. renal failure
    C. autosomal recessive inheritance
    D. occurrence primarily among ethnic groups originating from the Mediterranean area
    E. amyloidosis, which is felt to be a secondary phenomeonon

249

637. Children with sarcoidosis are more likely to be
   A. Caucasian
   B. urban
   C. more than ten years of age
   D. afebrile
   E. asymptomatic

638. Which of the following is known to be associated with the histiocytosis syndromes?
   A. Occurrence in males more common
   B. Malignancy
   C. Transmissible to animals
   D. Familial origin
   E. Occurrence of more disseminated lesions in older patients

639. The clinical type of histiocytosis with the highest mortality is
   A. Letterer–Siwe disease
   B. Hand–Schüller–Christian disease
   C. eosinophilic granuloma
   D. sarcoidosis
   E. none of the above are associated with significant mortality

640. Features of progeria include all of the following EXCEPT
   A. Short stature
   B. Sexual infantilism
   C. Little subcutaneous fat
   D. Hirsutism
   E. Aged appearance of facial features

DIRECTIONS: Each group of questions below consists of lettered headings, followed by a list of numbered words, phrases or statements. For each numbered word, phrase or statement, select the **one** lettered heading that is most closely associated with it. Each lettered heading may be selected once, more than once, or not at all.

A. Sarcoidosis
B. Histiocytosis
C. Both
D. Neither

641. Etiology believed to be viral

642. Skeleton most commonly involved tissue

643. Tissue biopsy critical for diagnosis

644. Steroids useful in treatment

645. Kveim test positive in active cases

DIRECTIONS: This section consists of situations, each followed by a series of questions. Study each situation, and select the **one** best answer to each question following it.

CASE 1 (Questions 646–650): You are in the emergency room at 6:30 A.M. preparing to admit an asthmatic who is in distress, when an ambulance arrives with an infant approximately four months old, who was found not breathing at home. Resuscitative efforts have thus far failed to elicit any response. You pronounce the infant dead, suspecting crib death.

646. True statements concerning this disorder include all of the following EXCEPT
   A. low birth weight is an important risk factor
   B. half of the infants have symptoms of a cold in the week prior to death
   C. after the first week of life, SIDS is the most important single cause of death of infants under one year of age
   D. viral studies are always indicated to confirm that a death was SIDS
   E. it has been reported to occur in infants who are only breastfed

647. True statements concerning the incidence of SIDS include each of the following EXCEPT
   A. the peak incidence of crib death is at five to six months
   B. the incidence is increased in lower socioeconomic classes
   C. it claims about 8000 babies a year in the United States
   D. the incidence is higher in females
   E. the incidence is increased among siblings of affected infants

648. The cause of sudden infant death in most cases is
   A. laryngospasm
   B. pulmonary aspiration of vomitus
   C. CNS hemorrhage
   D. pulmonary hemorrhage
   E. unknown

649. What percentage of infants dying suddenly will have some demonstrable lethal lesion at autopsy?

    A. 10%

    B. 15%

    C. 20%

    D. 25%

    E. 30%

650. Appropriate actions in this case include each of the following EXCEPT

    A. arrange for autopsy of the infant

    B. communicate information obtained about the cause of death as soon as possible

    C. designate sudden infant death syndrome on the death certificate, if indicated

    D. maintain contact with the parents for further counseling and support

    E. contacting the local police

Unclassified Disorders
Answers and Comments

635. E.   The syndrome occurs regardless of socioeconomic status, illegitimacy, or high parity in the mother. However, all of these factors significantly increase the risk, and males are more affected than females. The relationship to "spotting" in the first trimester has not been reported. (Ref. 2, p. 1770)

636. E.   This disease is classified as a primary amyloidosis because amyloid may be found very early in association with familial Mediterranean fever. (Ref. 2, p. 677)

637. C.   The disease is most common in rural communities and is uncommon in children less than ten years of age. (Ref. 2, p. 1776)

638. A.   Males are more common in all clinical groups and younger patients tend to have more disseminated lesions. (Ref. 2, p. 1777)

639. A.   These patients, because of their deep visceral involvement, have a significant mortality. (Ref. 2, p. 1777)

640. D.   Alopecia is generalized and frequently the skin is dry and wrinkled. (Ref. 2, p. 1776)

641. D.   Both histiocytosis and sarcoidosis have an unknown
642. B.   etiology, and steroids are useful in treatment, though
643. C.   the prognosis for both is very variable, and generally
644. C.   poor. Tissue biopsy is the best diagnostic tool, though
645. A.   the formation of a granuloma after injection of material from a sarcoid lesion is known as a positive Kveim test. The skeleton is most commonly affected in histiocytosis, with soft tissue organ involvement increasing as the spectrum of disease worsens. The lungs are most commonly affected in sarcoidosis, although hepatic and skin lesions, and uveitis are frequently found. (Ref. 2, pp. 1776, 1777)

646. D. Sudden infant death syndrome has no known etiology,
647. D. is associated with the risk factors mentioned, and is a
648. E. significant cause of death in the first year of life. About
649. B. 15% of infants dying suddenly will show some definable
650. E. cause at autopsy. Counseling and long-term support of
the family is essential. (Ref. 3, p. 748 and Ref. 2, p. 1770)

References

1. A.M. Rudolph and J.I.E. Hoffman, editors. *Pediatrics*, 17th edition. East Norwalk, CT: Appleton-Century-Crofts, 1982.

2. V.C. Vaughan, R.J. McKay, and R.E. Behrman. *Nelson Textbook of Pediatrics*. Philadelphia: W.B. Saunders Company, 1979.

3. S.S. Gillis and B.M. Kagan, editors. *Current Pediatric Therapy*. Philadelphia: W.B. Saunders Company, 1982.

257